STUDENT WORKBOOK FOR

ILLUSTRATED

Anatomy of the Head AND Neck

STUDENT WORKBOOK FOR

ILLUSTRATED

Anatomy of the Head AND Neck

SIXTH EDITION

MARGARET J. FEHRENBACH, RDH, MS

Oral Biologist and Dental Hygienist,
Adjunct Instructor, Bachelor of Applied Science Degree Dental Hygiene Program,
Seattle Central College, Seattle, Washington
Educational Consultant and Dental Science Technical Writer,
Seattle, Washington

ELSEVIER

Elsevier
3251 Riverport Lane
St. Louis, Missouri 63043

Notice

Practitioners and researchers must always rely on their own experience and knowledge in evaluating
and using any information, methods, compounds or experiments described herein. Because of rapid
advances in the medical sciences, in particular, independent verification of diagnoses and drug dosages
should be made. To the fullest extent of the law, no responsibility is assumed by Elsevier, authors, editors
or contributors for any injury and/or damage to persons or property as a matter of products liability,
negligence or otherwise, or from any use or operation of any methods, products, instructions, or ideas
contained in the material herein.

Content Strategist: Joslyn Dumas/Kelly Skelton
Content Development Director: Laurie Gower
Content Development Specialist: Brooke Kannady
Publishing Services Manager: Shereen Jameel
Senior Project Manager: Kamatchi Madhavan
Cover Designer: Gopalakrishnan Venkatraman

Printed in India

Last digit is the print number: 9 8 7 6 5 4 3 2

Working together
to grow libraries in
developing countries

www.elsevier.com • www.bookaid.org

PREFACE

This new companion to *Illustrated Anatomy of the Head and Neck* provides a wide range of activities and skill-building exercises to strengthen the student dental professional's understanding of the principles discussed in the main textbook. This Workbook features activities related to each chapter of the text, such as structure identification exercises, glossary exercises, and review questions. Also included is an exercise in patient examination procedures for both extraoral and intraoral structures in order to integrate clinical information with basic science information. Summary case studies are also included, as well as updated removable flashcards using the latest original illustrations from the textbook.

Additional material for students can be found online on the associated Evolve website, including answers to the Workbook's glossary exercises, review questions, and case studies by way of the instructor(s). We hope that this material will help students integrate their knowledge more easily into clinical dental coursework.

Margaret J. Fehrenbach, RDH, MS

CONTENTS

Note: Answers can be obtained from comparing your fill-ins to the labels on numbered figures from the textbook. Feel free to add additional labeling as needed as well as other notations.

Chapter 1: Introduction to Head and Neck Anatomy

1. Fig. 1.3

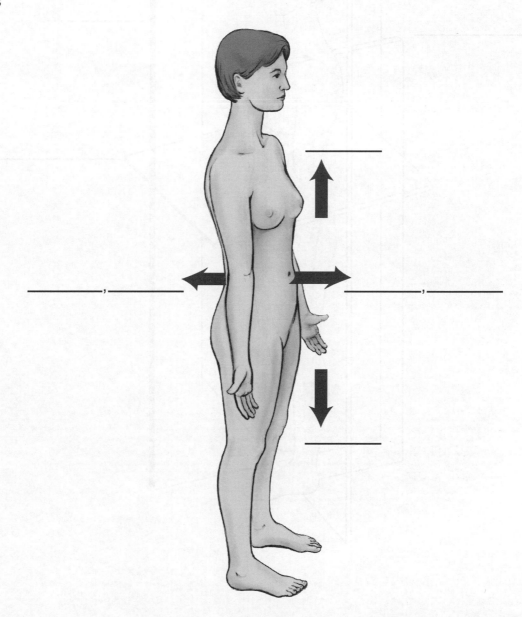

_____

_____ , _____   _____ , _____

_____

2. Fig. 1.4

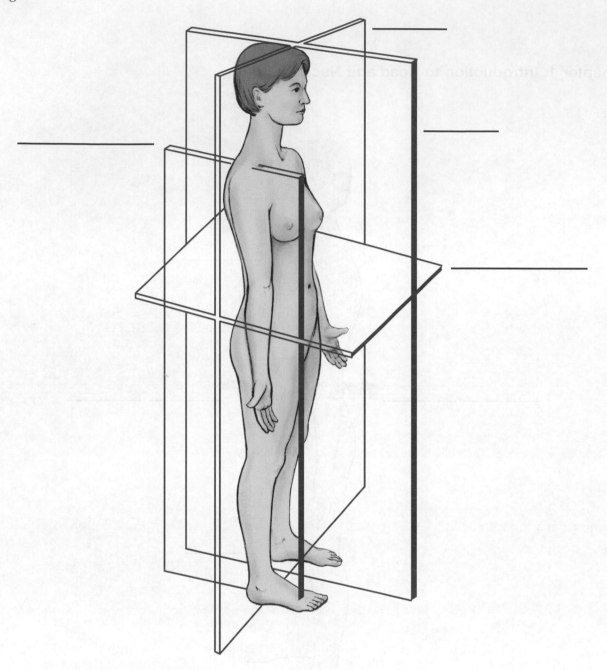

3. Fig. 1.5

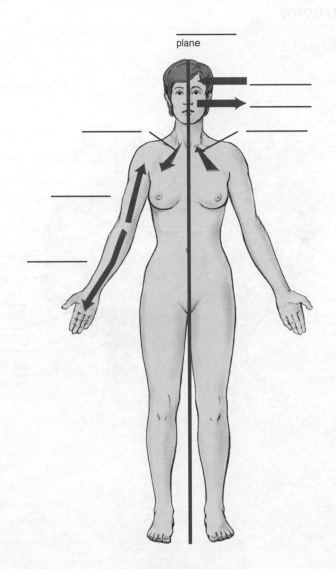

plane

4. Fig. 1.6

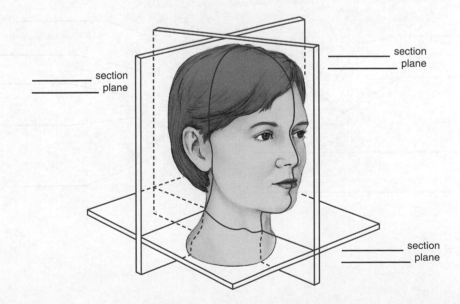

section plane

section plane

section plane

Chapter 2: Surface Anatomy

1. Figs. 2.1, 2.2, *A*, 2.4, 2.6, 2.7, and 2.9

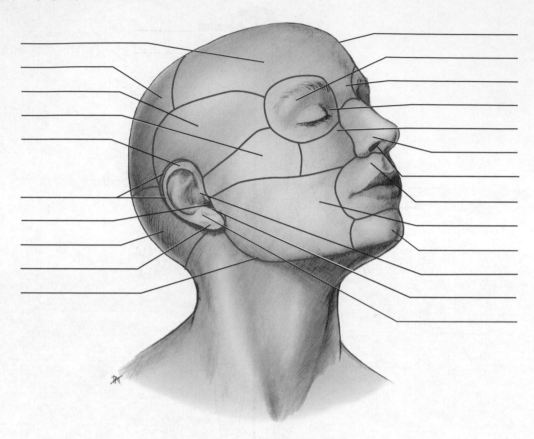

2. Fig. 2.6, *A*

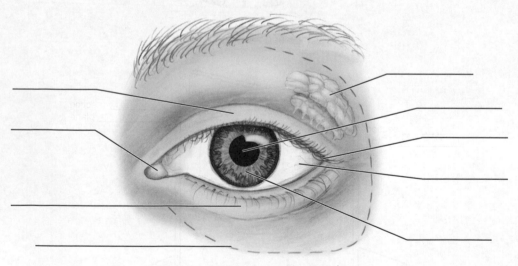

3. Fig. 2.11 (From Fehrenbach MJ and Popowics *T. Illustrated dental embryology, histology, and anatomy,* 5th ed., Elsevier, St. Louis, 2020.)

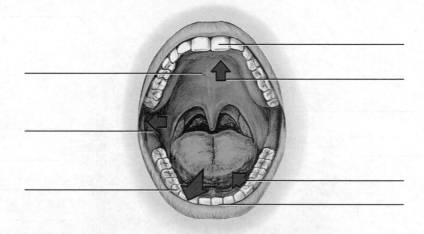

4. Fig. 2.17, *A* (From Fehrenbach MJ and Popowics *T. Illustrated dental embryology, histology, and anatomy,* 5th ed., Elsevier, St. Louis, 2020.)

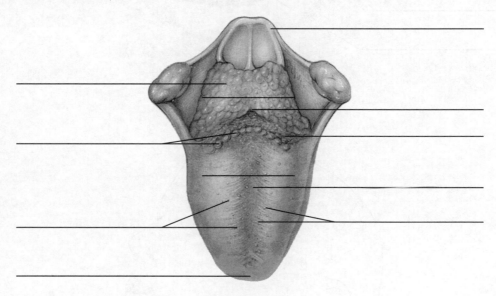

5. Fig. 2.20

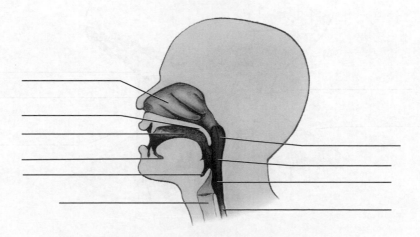

6. Fig. 2.21

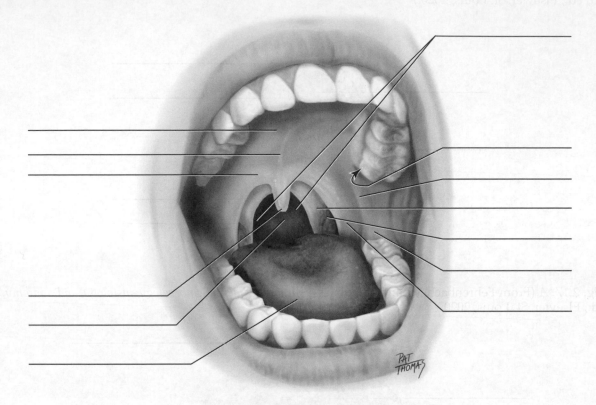

7. Fig. 2.23

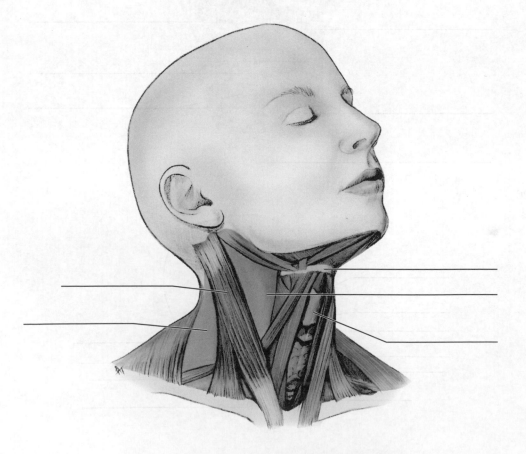

8. Fig. 2.25

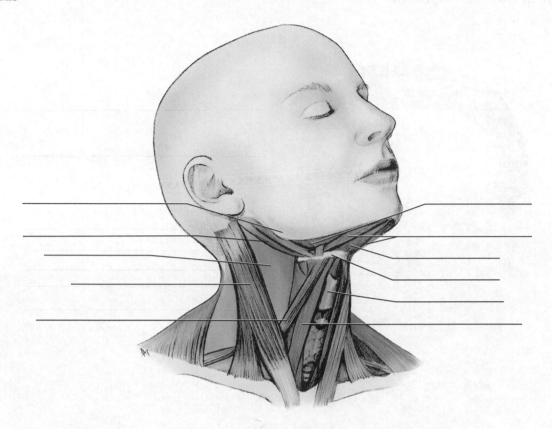

9. Fig. 2.26

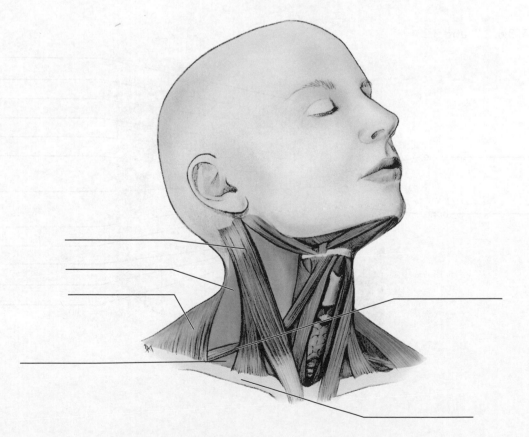

Chapter 3: Skeletal System

1. Fig. 3.4

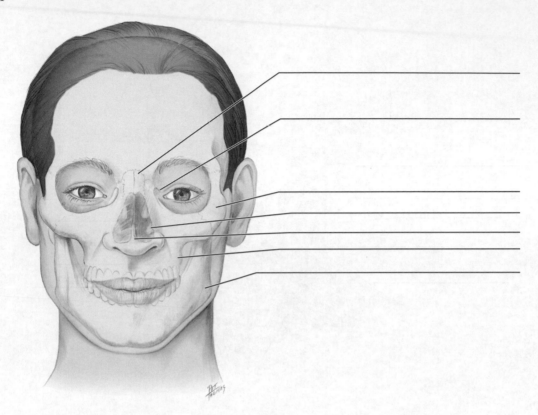

2. Figs. 3.5, 3.6, 3.7, and 3.23

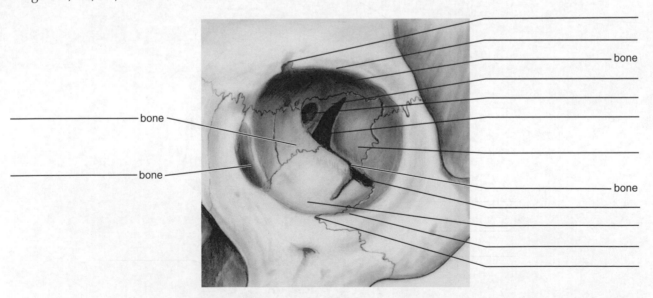

bone

bone

bone

bone

bone

3. Figs. 3.20, 3.23, and 3.27

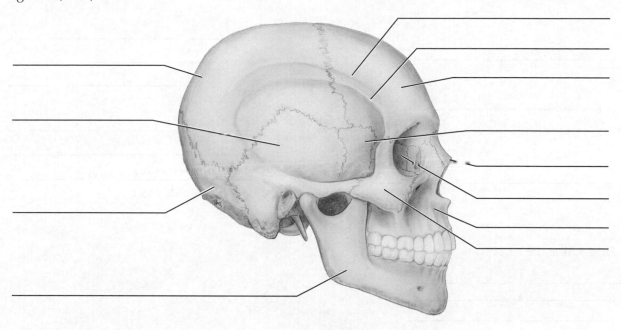

4. Fig. 3.22, *A*

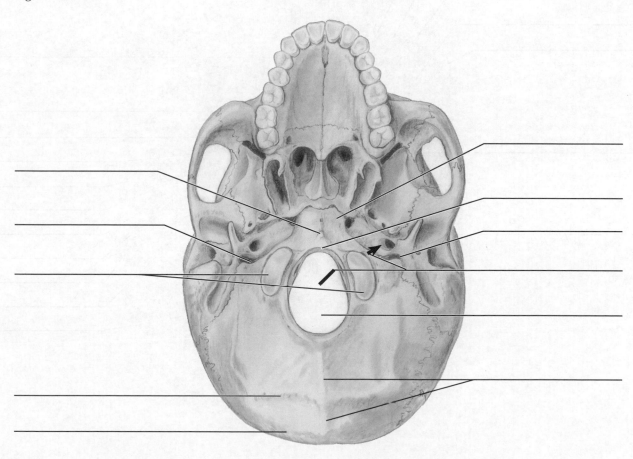

5. Figs. 3.28, 3.29, and 3.30

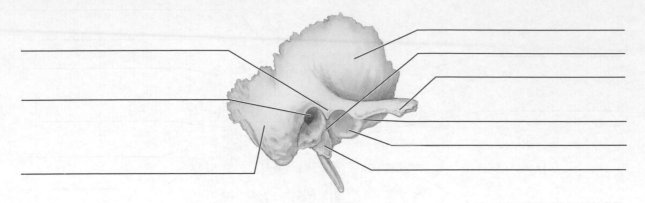

6. Figs. 3.31 and 3.32, *A*

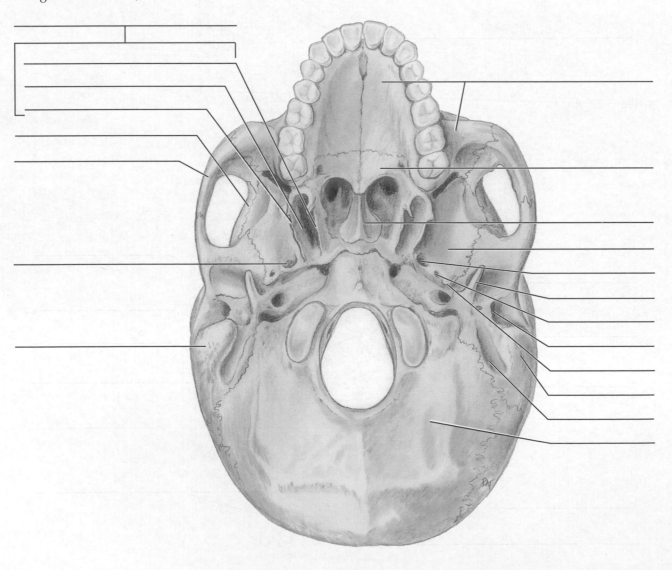

7. Fig. 3.33, *A*

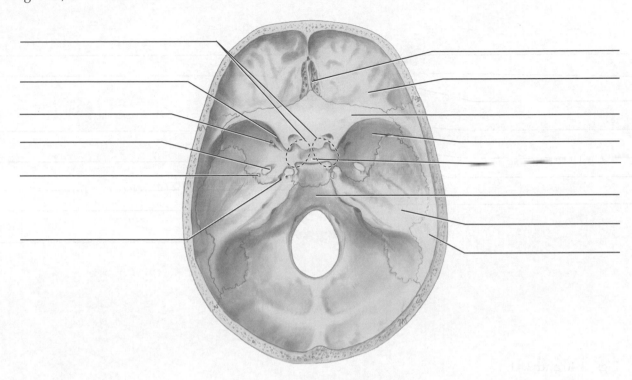

8. Fig. 3.35, *A*

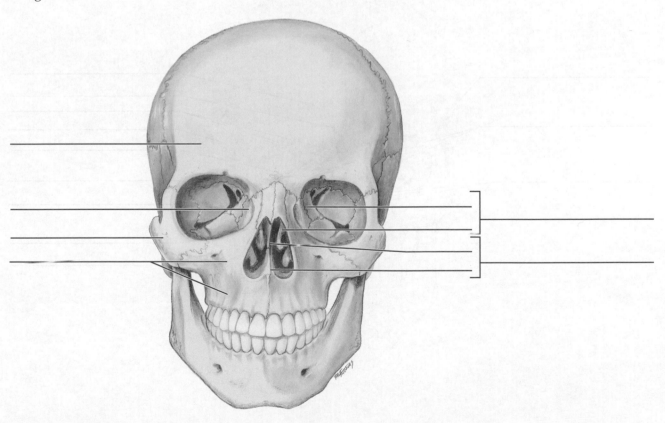

9. Fig. 3.38

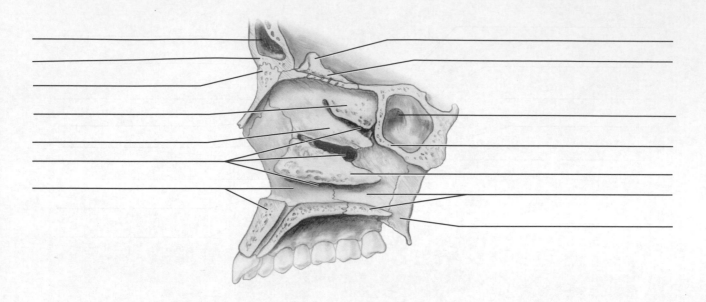

10. Figs. 3.40 and 3.41

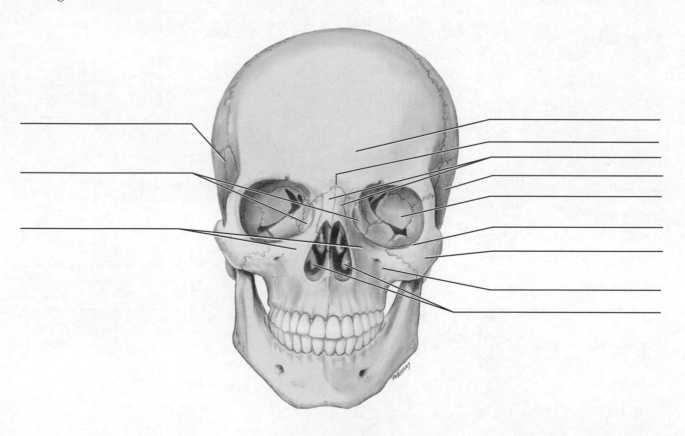

11. Fig. 3.42, *A*

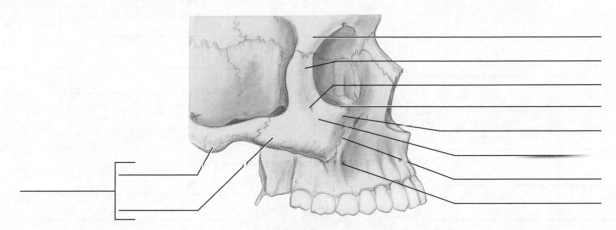

12. Fig. 3.44, *A*

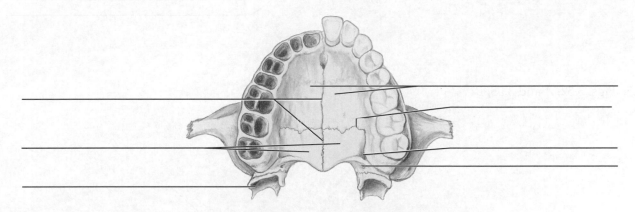

13. Fig. 3.45

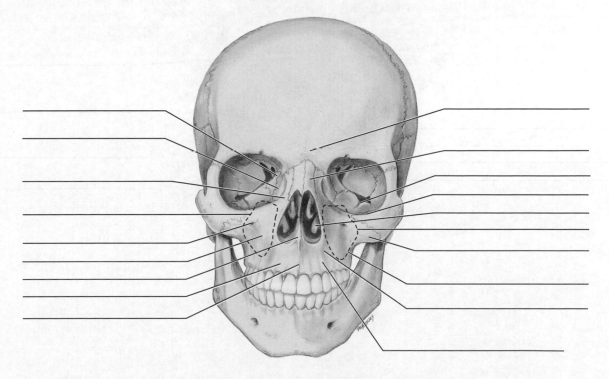

14. Fig. 3.47, *A*

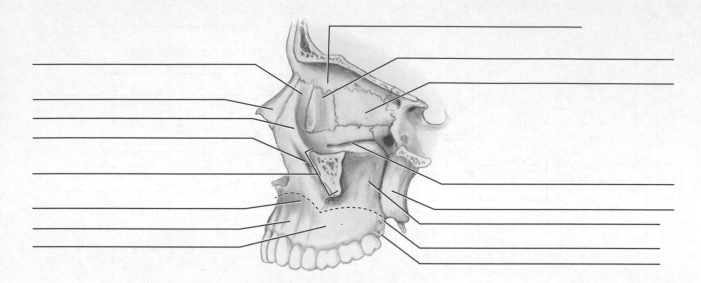

15. Figs. 3.52, *A* and 3.55, *B*

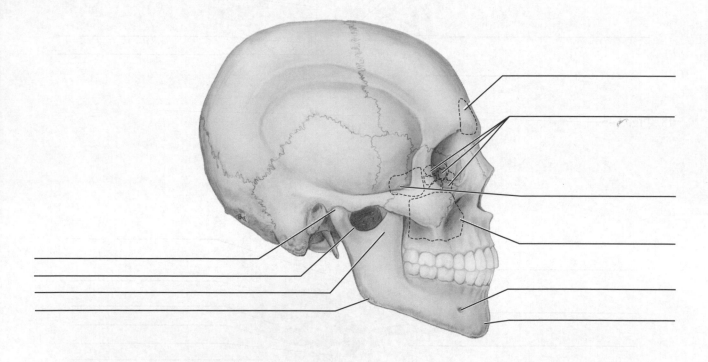

16. Fig. 3.60

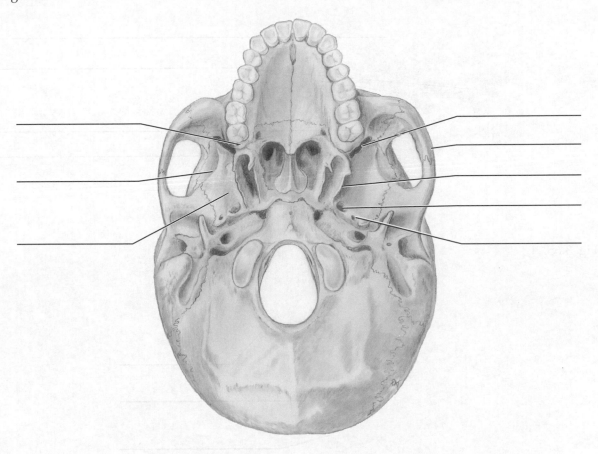

17. Fig. 3.61

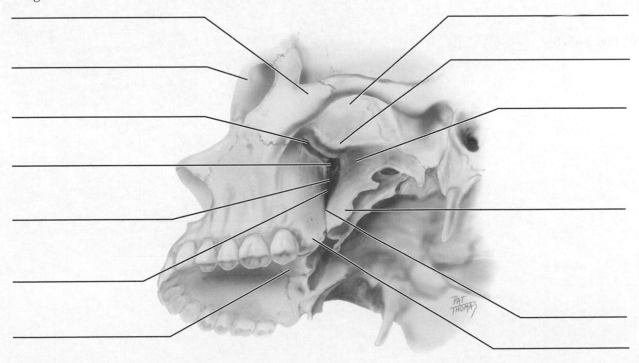

18. Fig. 3.62

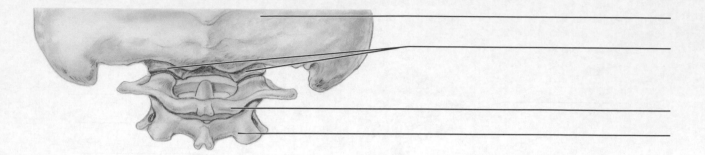

19. Fig. 3.65, *A*

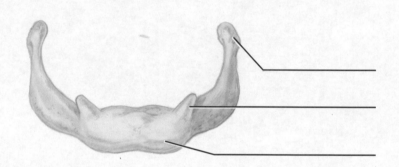

20. Fig. 3.65, *B*

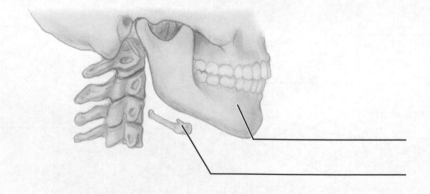

Chapter 4: Muscular System

1. Fig. 4.4, *A*

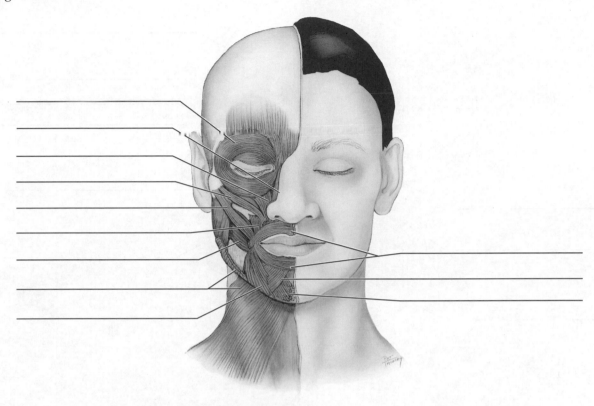

2. Fig. 4.4, *B*

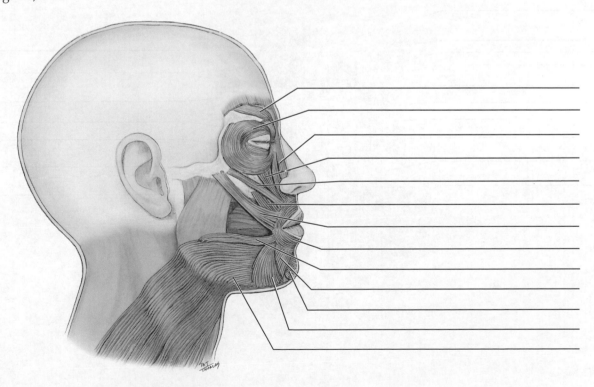

3. Figs. 4.22 and 4.23

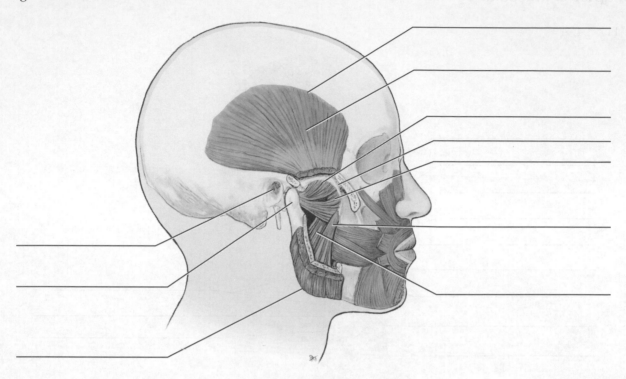

4. Fig. 4.24

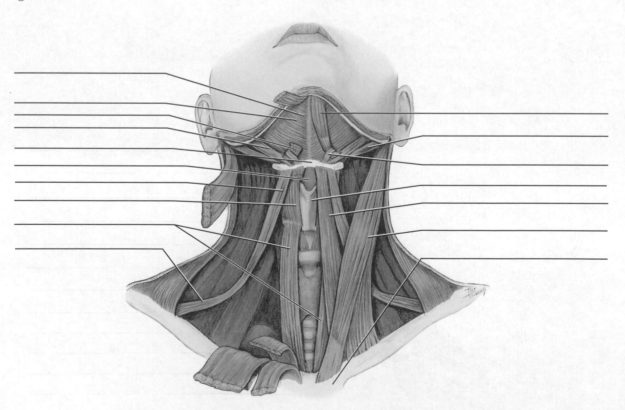

5. Figs. 4.25 and 4.27

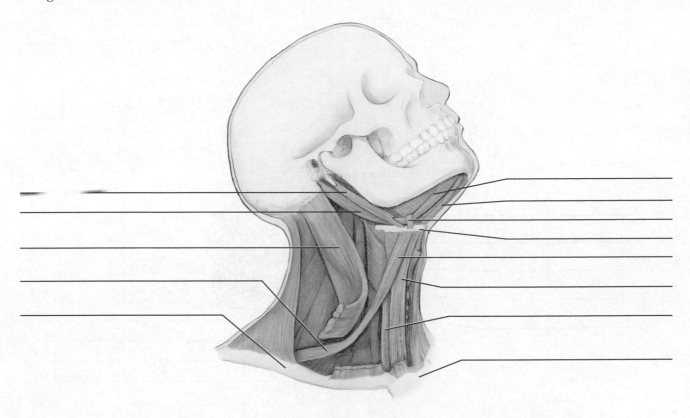

6. Fig. 4.28, *A*

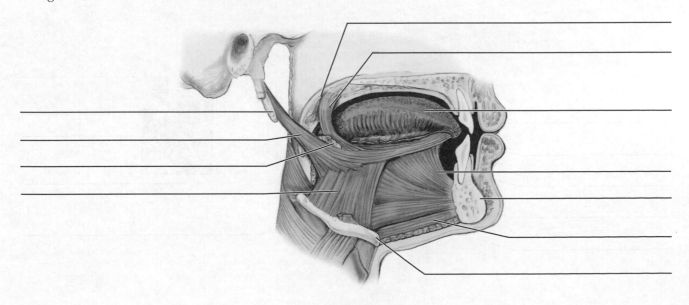

7. Fig. 4.29, *B*

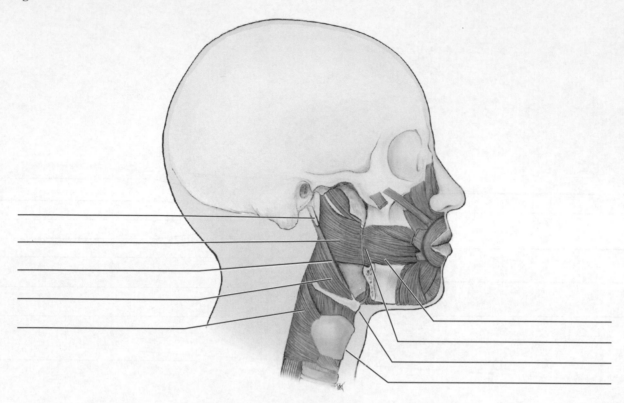

8. Fig. 4.30

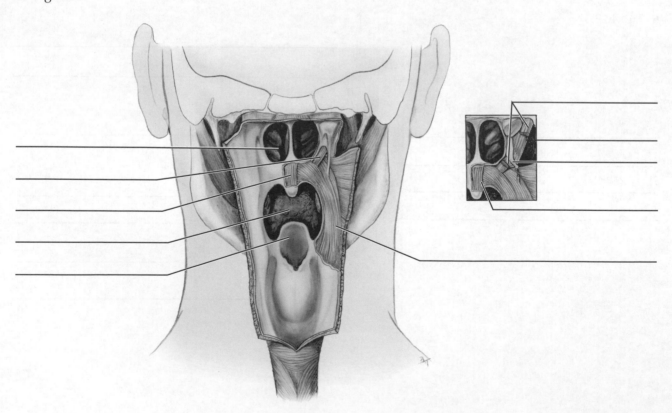

Chapter 5: Temporomandibular Joint

1. Figs. 5.1, *A*, 5.2, and 5.4, *A* and *B*

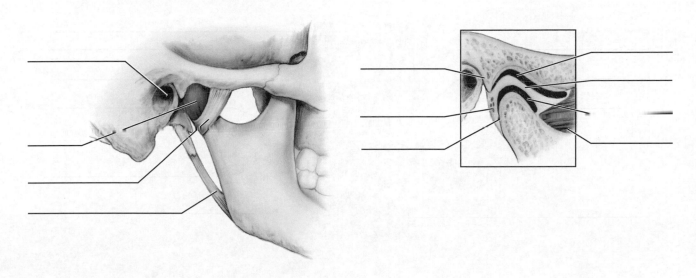

2. Figs. 5.3 and 5.5

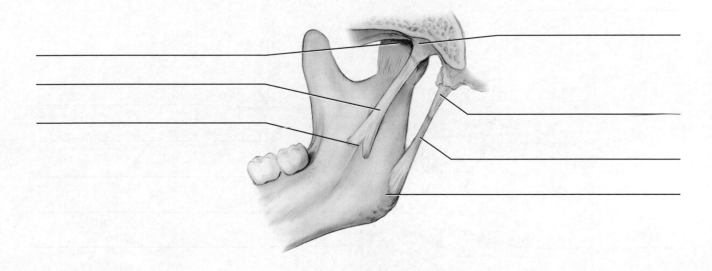

Chapter 6: Vascular System

1. Fig. 6.1

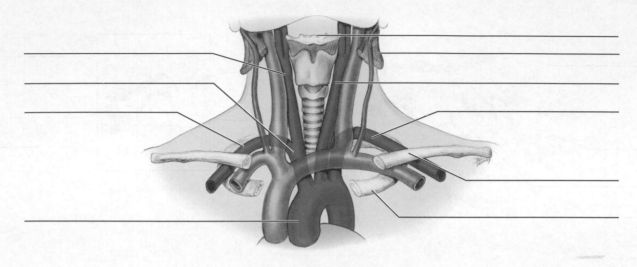

2. Fig. 6.3, *A*

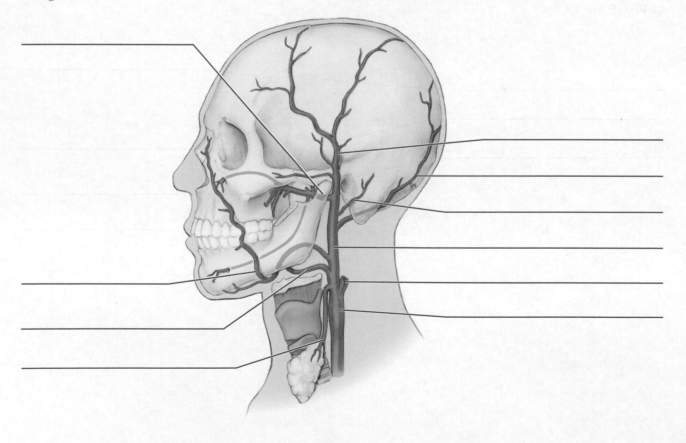

3. Fig. 6.5

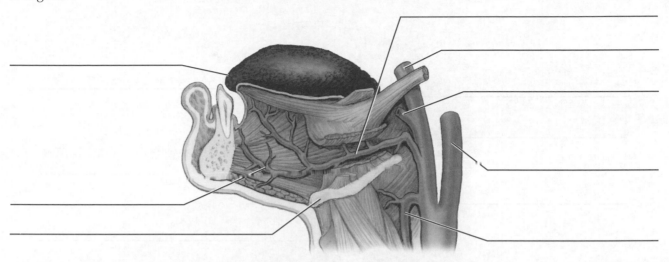

4. Fig. 6.6

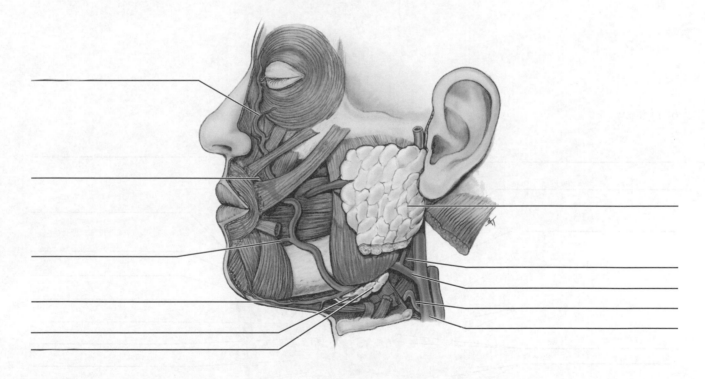

5. Fig. 6.8

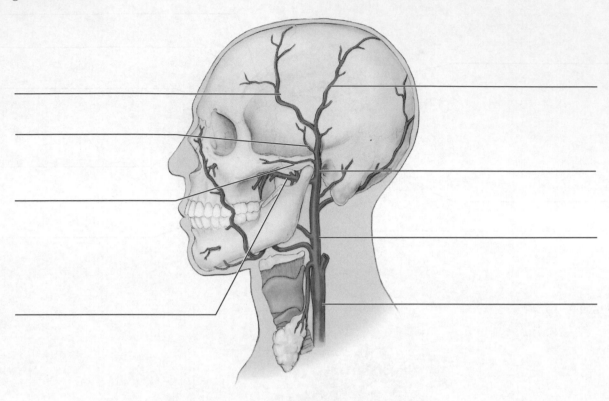

6. Fig. 6.9

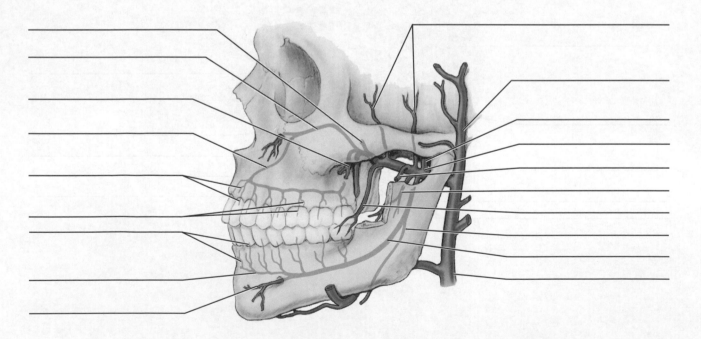

7. Fig. 6.11

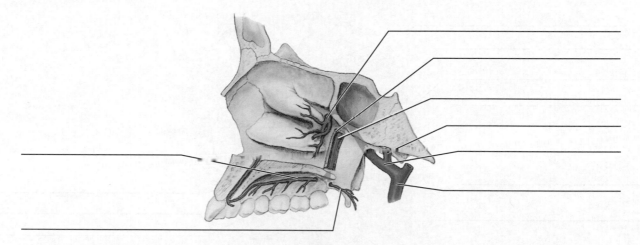

8. Fig. 6.12

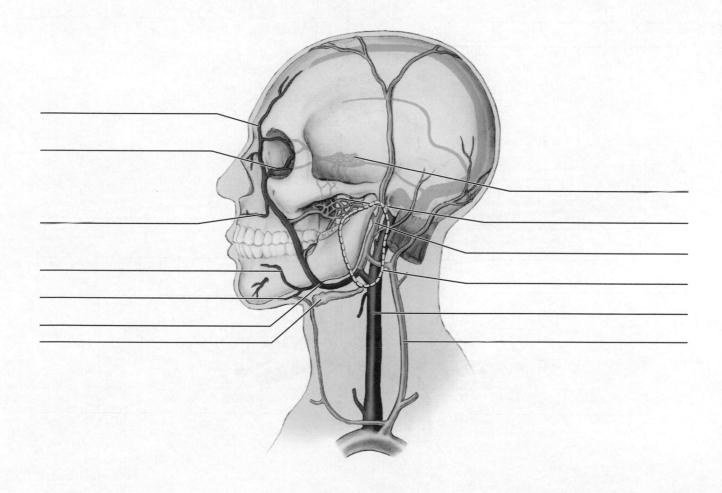

9. Fig. 6.13

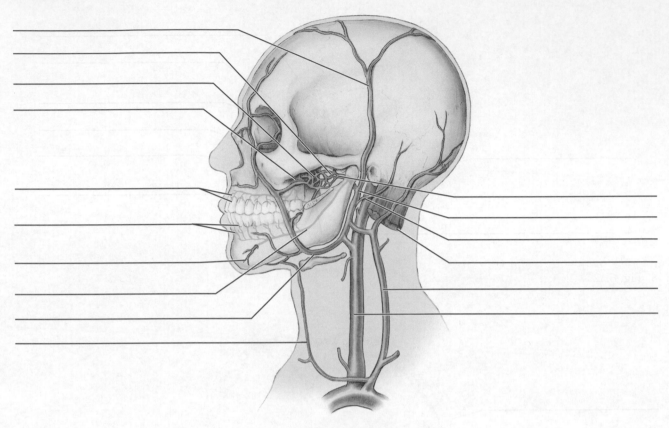

10. Fig. 6.14

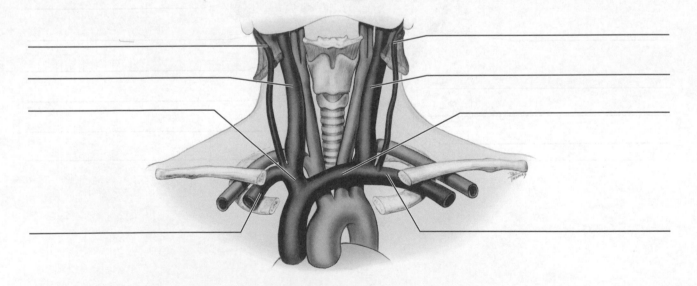

Chapter 7: Glandular Tissue

1. Fig. 7.1

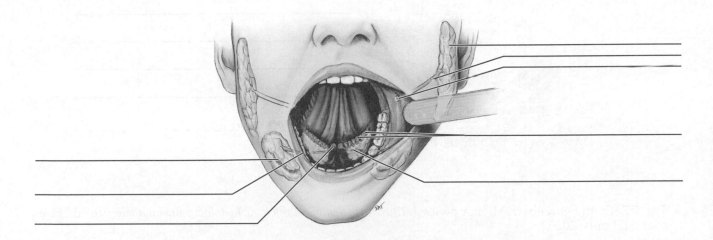

2. Fig. 7.2

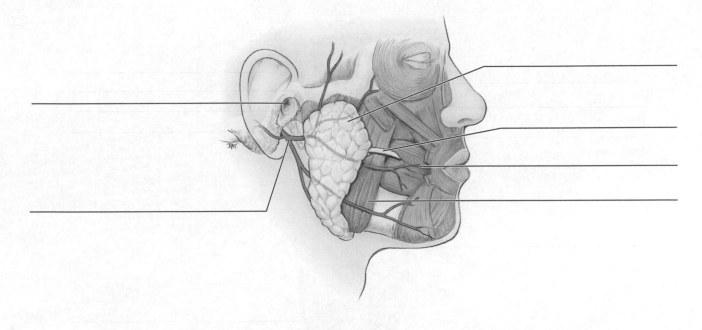

3. Fig. 7.5

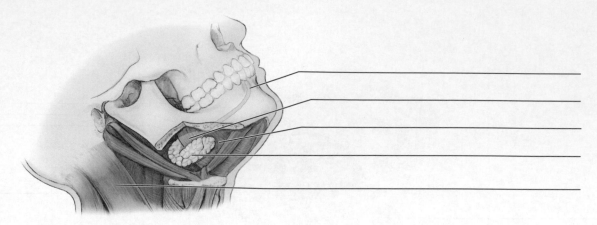

4. Fig. 7.7 (From Fehrenbach MJ, Popowics T: *Illustrated dental embryology, histology, and anatomy,* 5th ed., Elsevier, St. Louis, 2020.)

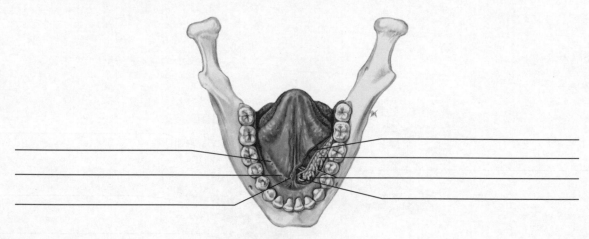

5. Fig. 7.11, *A*

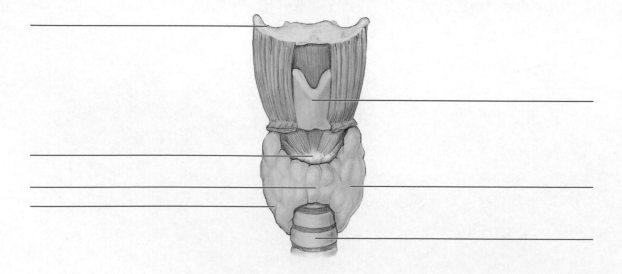

6. Fig. 7.14

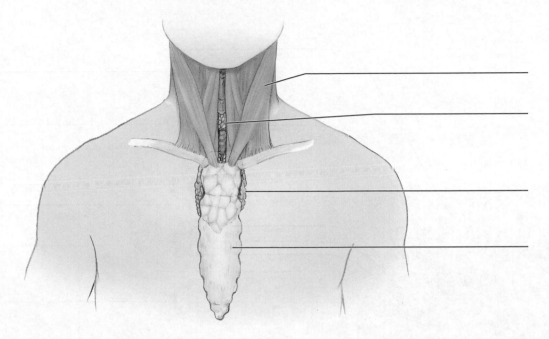

Chapter 8: Nervous System

1. Fig. 8.4, *A*

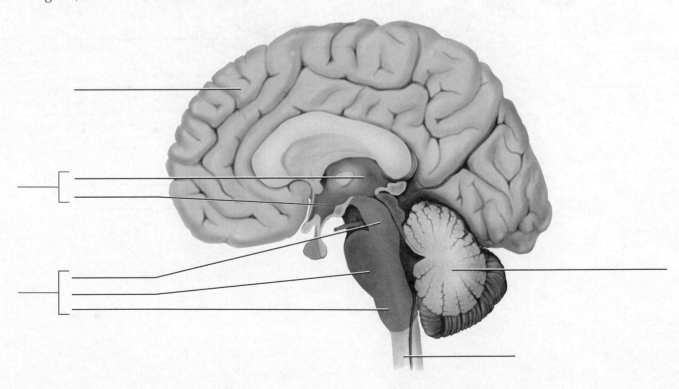

2. Fig. 8.5

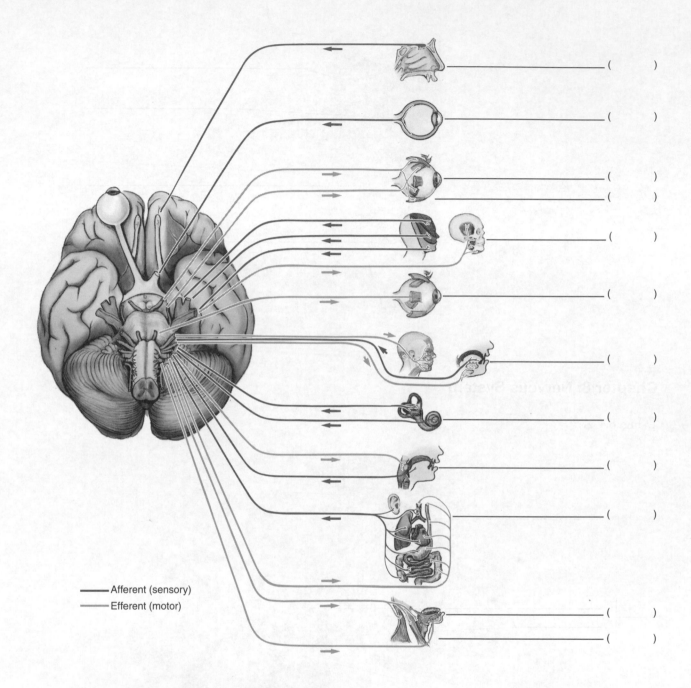

Afferent (sensory)
Efferent (motor)

3. Fig. 8.6

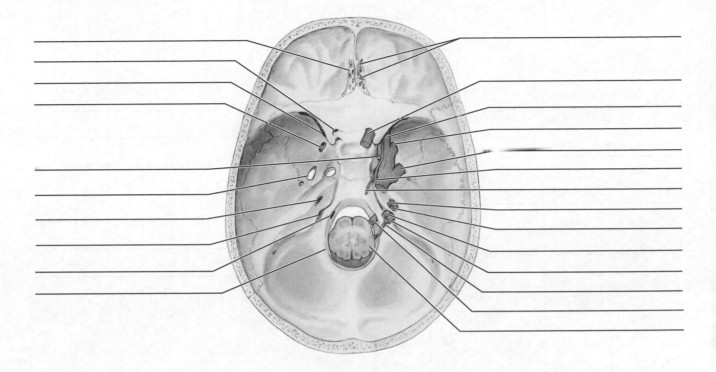

4. Figs. 8.8 and 8.11

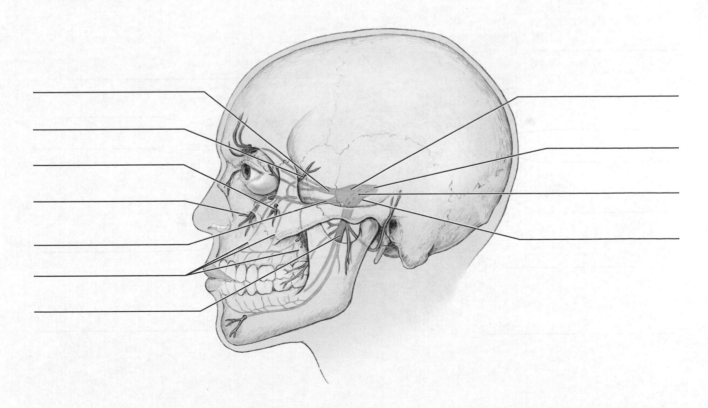

5. Fig. 8.13

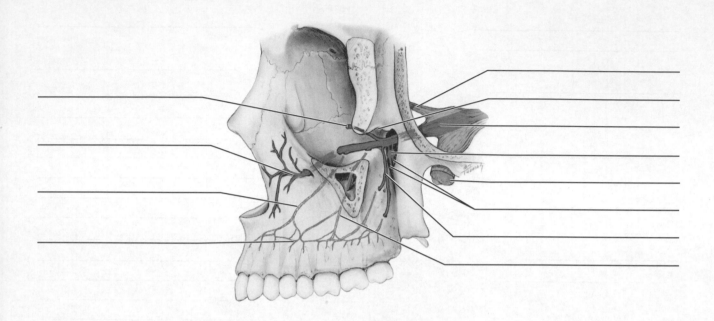

6. Fig. 8.14, *A*

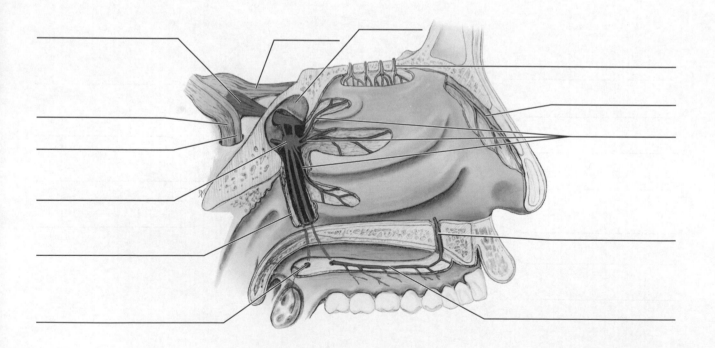

7. Fig. 8.18, *A*

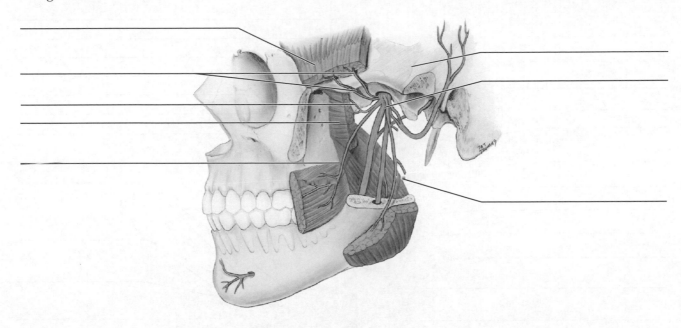

8. Fig. 8.19, *A*

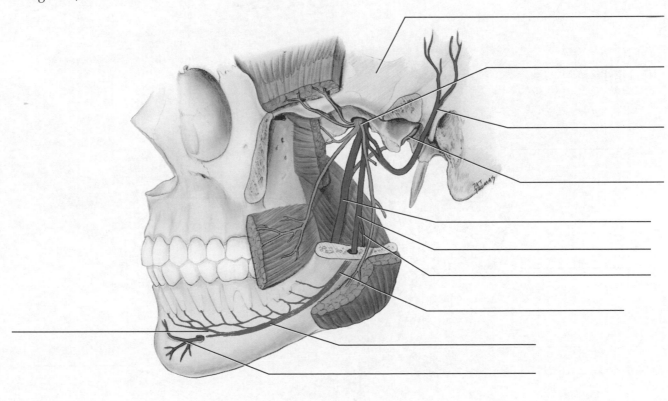

9. Fig. 8.20

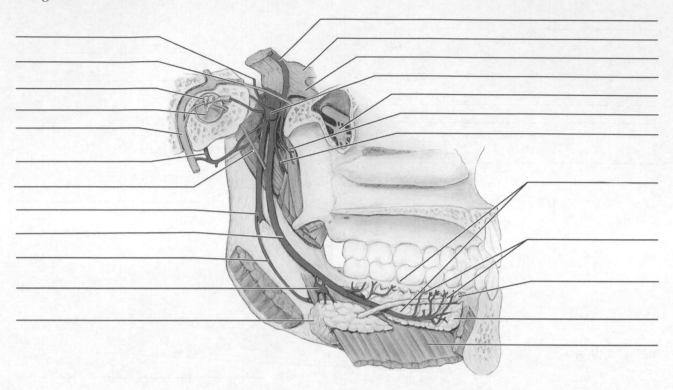

10. Fig. 8.21

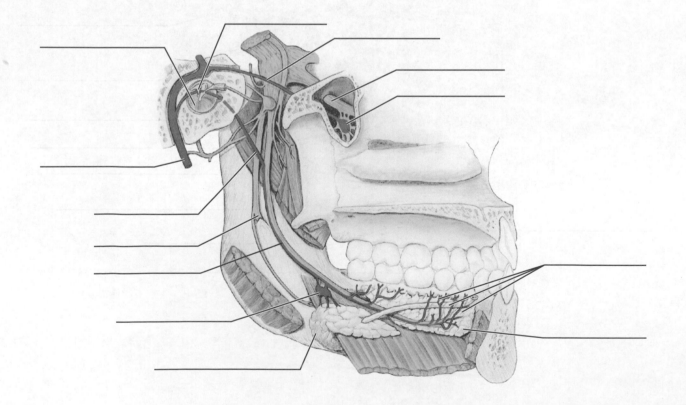

Chapter 9: Anatomy of Local Anesthesia

1. Fig. 9.7

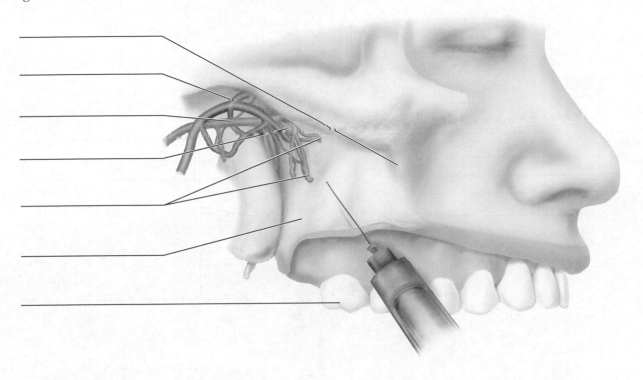

2. Fig. 9.37

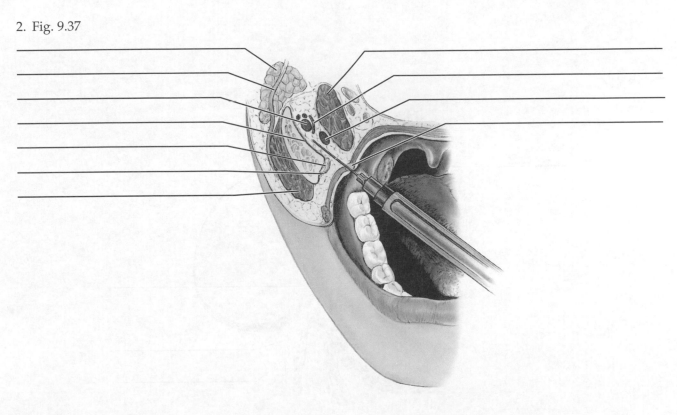

Chapter 10: Lymphatic System

1. Fig. 10.1

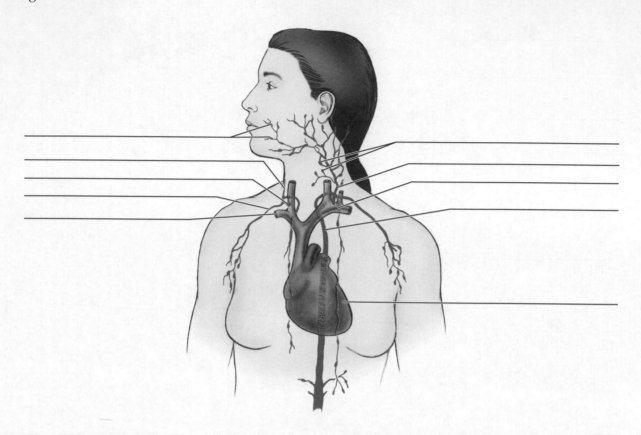

2. Fig. 10.2

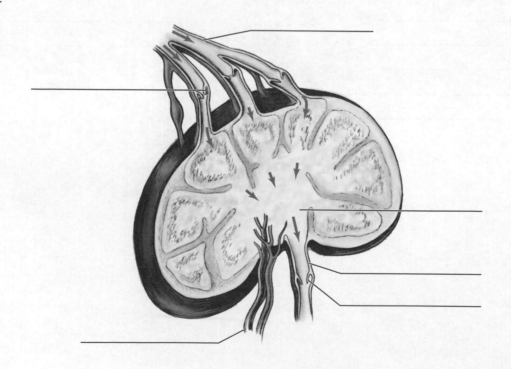

3. Fig. 10.3

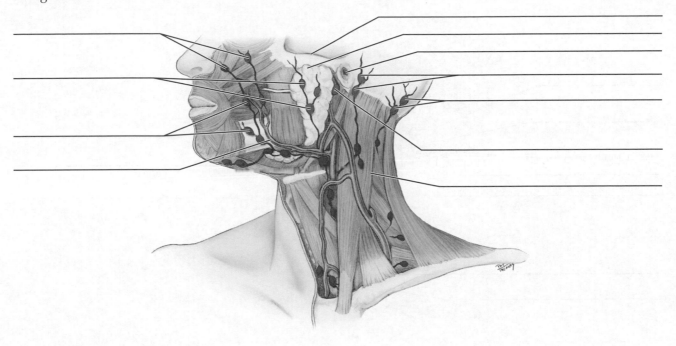

4. Fig. 10.7

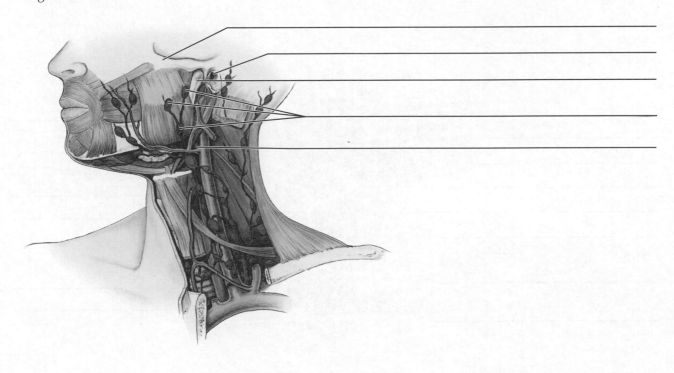

5. Fig. 10.10

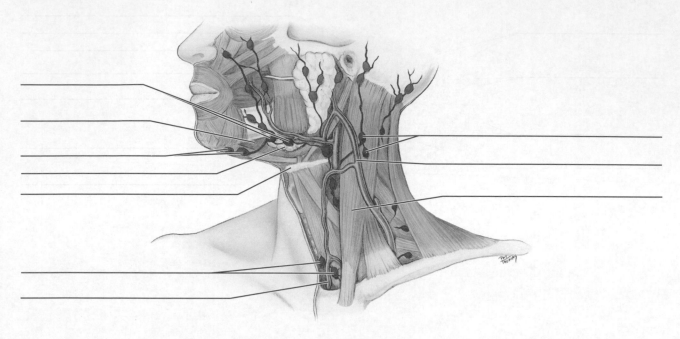

6. Fig. 10.15

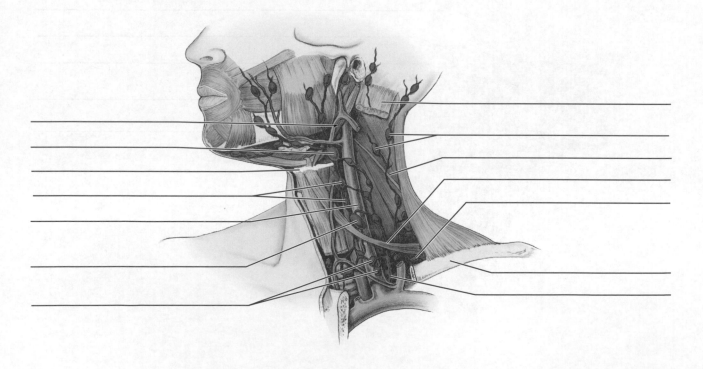

7. Fig. 10.21, *A*

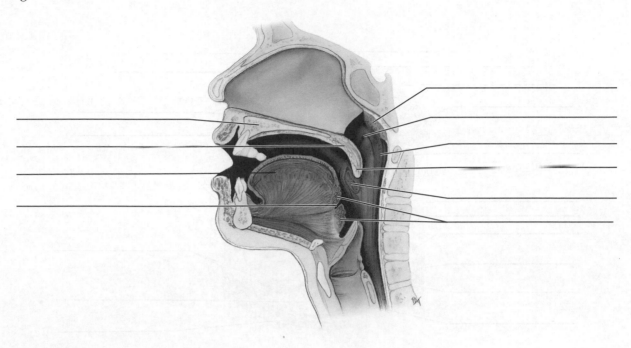

Chapter 11: Fasciae and Spaces

1. Fig. 11.1, *A*

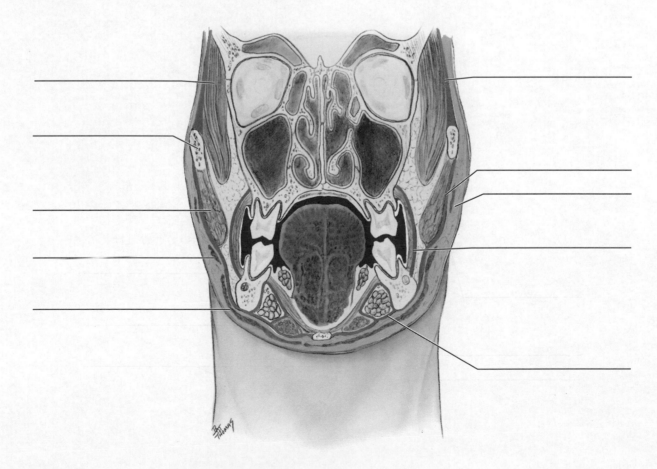

2. Fig. 11.1, *B*

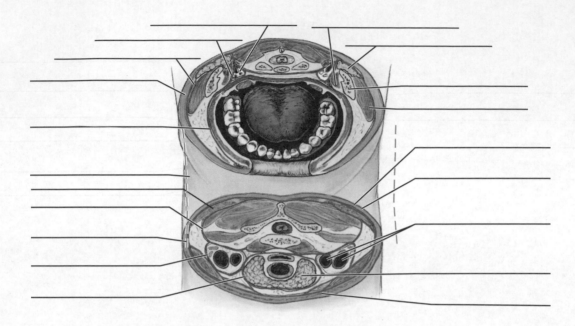

3. Fig. 11.2

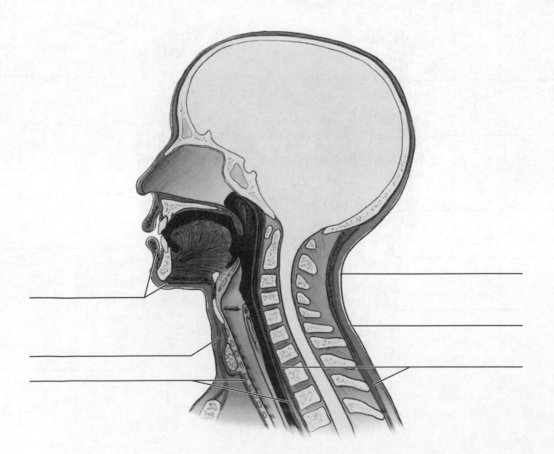

4. Fig. 11.3

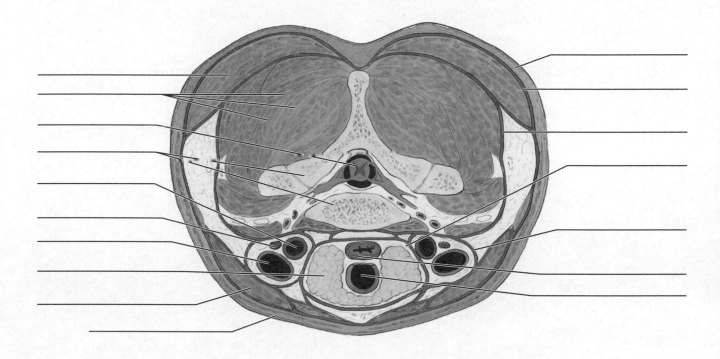

5. Fig. 11.4

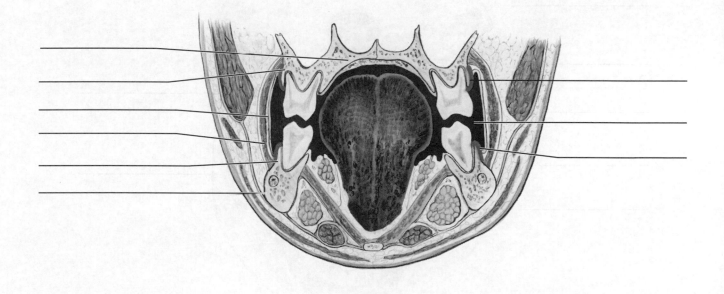

6. Fig. 11.5

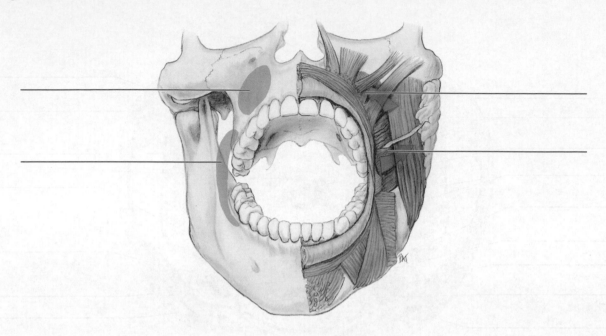

7. Fig. 11.6

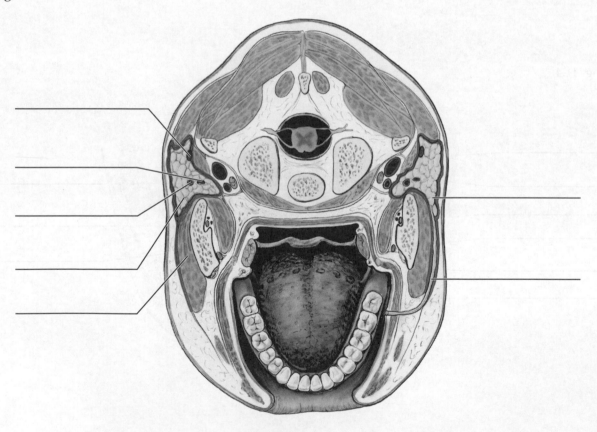

8. Fig. 11.7

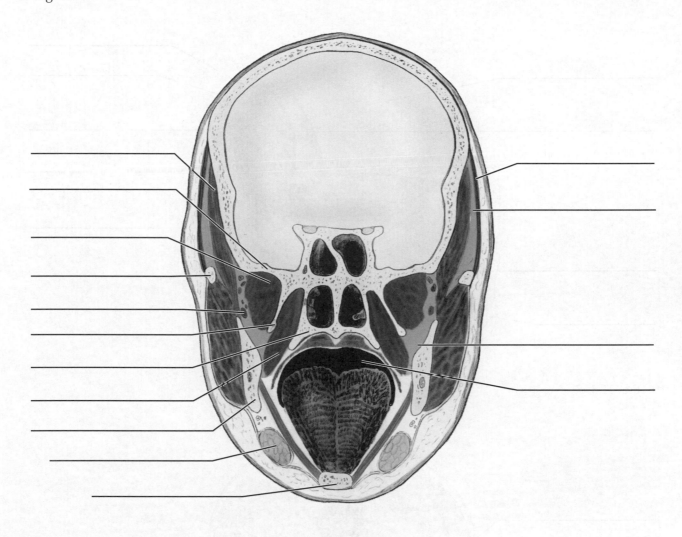

9. Fig. 11.8, *A*

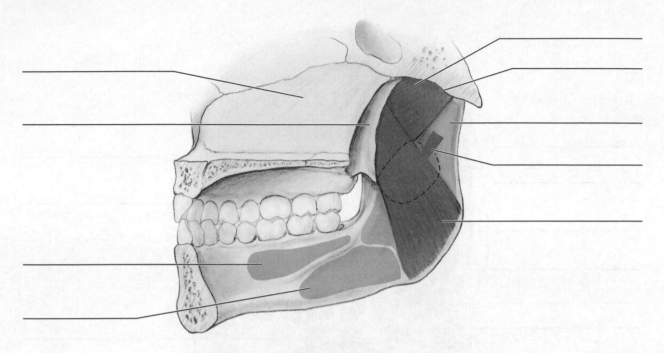

10. Fig. 11.8, *B*

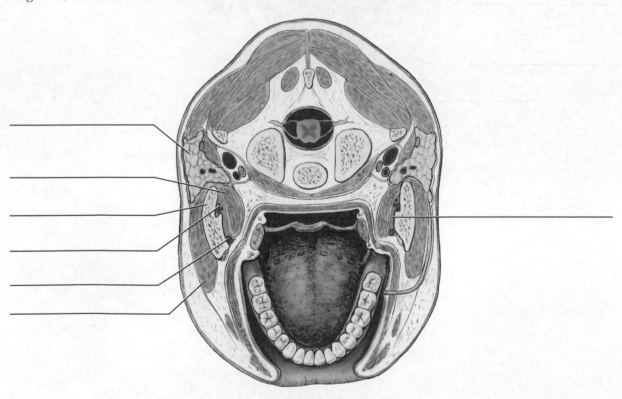

11. Fig. 11.9

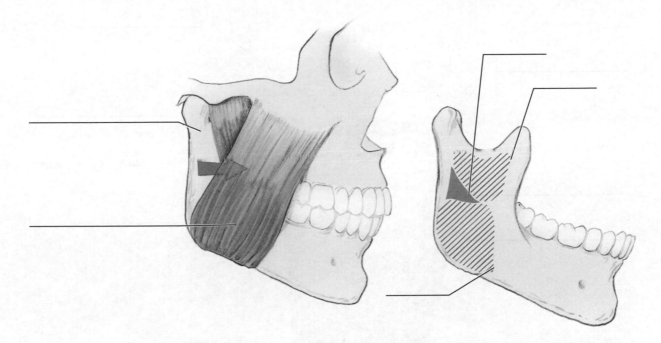

12. Fig. 11.10, *A*

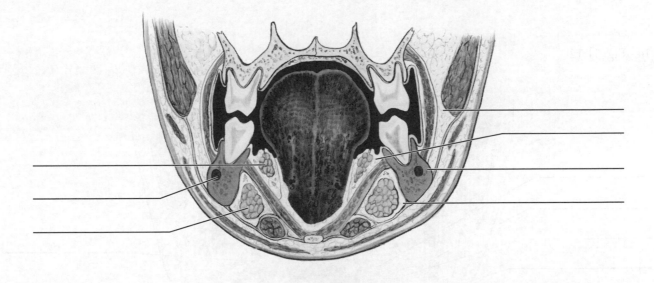

13. Fig. 11.11

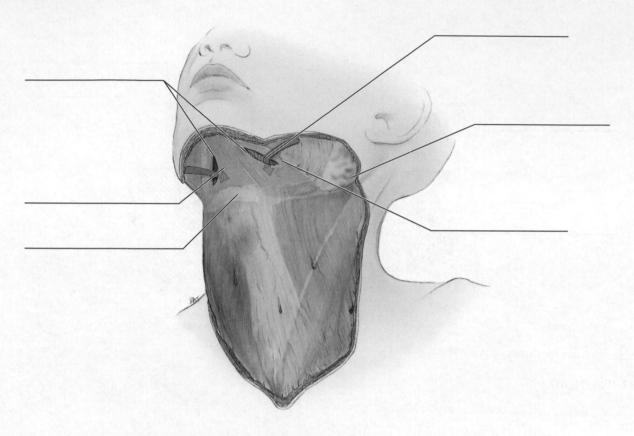

14. Fig. 11.12

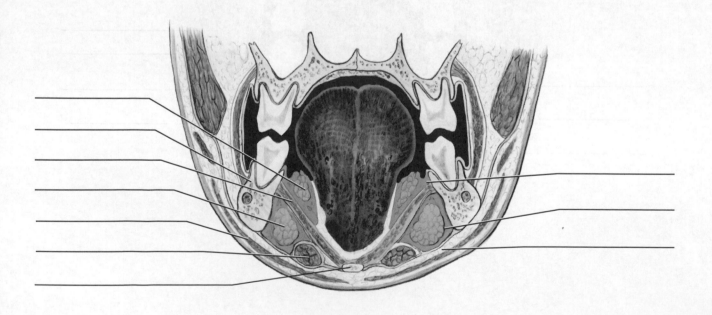

16. Fig. 11.13, *A*

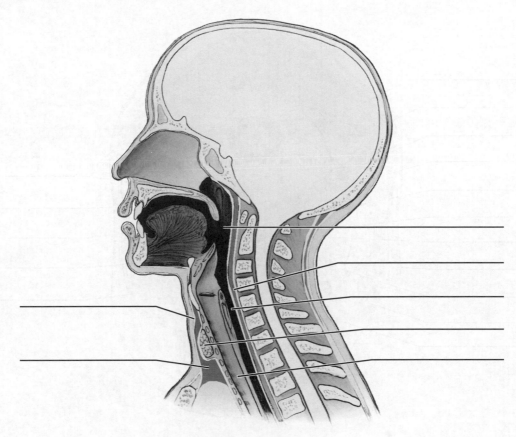

17. Fig. 11.13, *B*

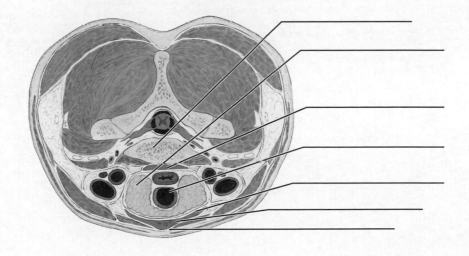

15. Fig. 11.14

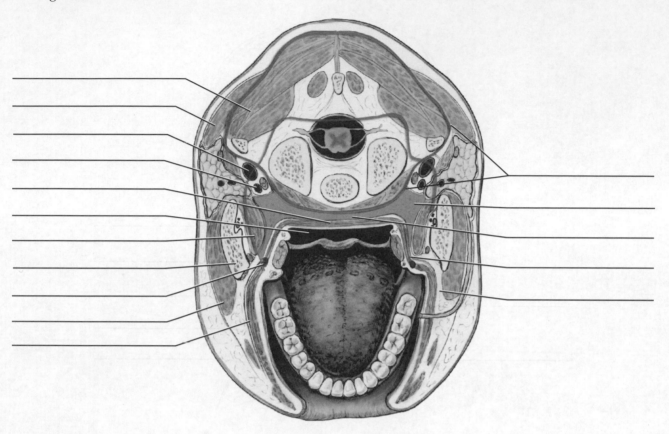

Basic Clinical Supplies Needed: The student dental professional will need the following basic supplies for the clinical examination exercises: dental chair and light, mirror instrument, hand mirror, and workbook-included form. Standard infection control precautions, including personal protection equipment, must be adhered to as outlined by the Occupational Safety and Health Administration Bloodborne Pathogens Standard.

Initial Procedural Steps: After completing the medical and dental history and review, the patient should be seated in a dental chair, either supine or upright as needed. Use preprocedural antimicrobial mouthrinse, remove any pigmented lipsticks, and apply nonpetroleum lubricant to dry lips; ask to take out any removable prostheses. Good lighting and exposure of the area being assessed are essential (e.g., collar and tie loosened, personal glasses removed).

Explanations of the reasons for performing extraoral and intraoral examinations for the patient and their relationship of these examinations to dental treatment as well as importance of self-examination, including the terms used in these examinations, are discussed in the associated textbook. Within the associated textbook's **Appendix B** is more specific information on extraoral and intraoral clinical examination skills, including methods of palpation. Within the associated textbook's **Appendix C** is a table of clinical photographs related to each of the steps as well a discussion of typical findings. Any more in-depth examination of these areas can be done in the future by student dental professionals after additional coursework in oral pathology, periodontology, dental materials, radiology, and clinical rotations or using references in bibliography within the associated textbook's **Appendix A**.

Part 1: CLINICAL EXAMINATION EXERCISE: Extraoral Examination Procedure

Directions: During this exercise of an extraoral examination procedure, identify any atypical findings by using both visual inspection and palpation during the examination. Make sure to note any of these atypical findings such as with traumatic injury, if applicable. Include specific location using nearby structures. Also note any abnormal findings; if found, take nonidentifiable clinical photographs to be shared (after being granted permission) with other students and make appropriate referrals. Include also any palpable lymph nodes of the face and neck, if applicable. See the associated textbook's **Appendix C** for discussion on what constitutes an atypical or abnormal finding.

Regions	Steps	Findings
Overall evaluation of the face, head, and neck, including the skin	• Visually observe symmetry and coloration of the face and neck with patient sitting upright and relaxed, while allowing the patient to look at a hand mirror throughout so as to understand the steps for self-examination.	
Frontal region, including forehead and frontal sinuses	• Visually inspect and bilaterally palpate the forehead including the frontal sinuses.	
Parietal and occipital regions including scalp, hair, and occipital lymph nodes	• Visually inspect the entire scalp by moving the hair, especially around the hairline, starting from one ear and proceeding to the other ear. • Then bilaterally palpate the occipital lymph nodes on each side of the base of the head while the patient leans the head forward.	

(Continued)

Regions	Steps	Findings
Temporal and auricular regions, including scalp, ears, and auricular lymph nodes	• Visually inspect and manually palpate the external ear as well as the scalp, face, and auricular lymph nodes around each ear.	
Orbital regions, including the eyes	• Visually inspect the eyes with their movements and responses to light and action.	
Nasal region, including the nose	• Visually inspect and bilaterally palpate the external nose, starting at the root of the nose and proceeding to its apex.	
Infraorbital and zygomatic regions, including the muscles of facial expressions, facial lymph nodes, maxillae, maxillary sinuses, and temporomandibular joints (TMJs)	• Visually inspect inferior to the orbits, especially noting the use of the muscles of facial expression. • Visually inspect and bilaterally palpate each side of the face and facial lymph nodes, moving from the infraorbital region to the labial commissure and then to the surface of the mandible. • Visually inspect and bilaterally palpate the maxillary sinuses. • Ask to open and close the mouth several times. Then ask to move the opened lower jaw left, then right, and then forward. Ask if there is any pain or tenderness experienced and note any sounds made by either joint. • To further access the TMJs, gently place a finger into the outer part of each external acoustic meatus during these movements.	
Buccal regions, including the masseter muscles, parotid salivary glands, and mandible	• Visually inspect and bilaterally palpate the masseter and parotid gland by starting in anterior to each ear, moving to the zygomatic arch, and then inferior to the angle of the mandible. • Then place the fingers of each hand over each masseter and ask to clench the teeth together several times.	
Mental region, including the chin	• Visually inspect and bilaterally palpate the chin.	

Regions	Steps	Findings
Submandibular and submental triangles, including submandibular and sublingual salivary glands and associated lymph nodes	• While asking to lower the chin, manually palpate the submandibular and sublingual glands as well as the associated lymph nodes underneath the chin and on the inferior border of the mandible. • Then push the tissue in the area over the bony inferior border of the mandible on each side, where it is grasped and rolled.	
Anterior and posterior cervical triangles, including sternocleidomastoid (SCM) muscles and associated cervical nodes	• Manually palpate on each side of the neck the superficial cervical nodes while asking to look straight ahead, starting inferior to the ear and continuing the whole length of the SCM muscles surface to the clavicles. • Then ask to tilt the head to the one side and then to the other to allow palpation of the superior deep cervical lymph nodes on the underside of the anterior and posterior aspects of the SCM muscles as before. • Then ask to raise the shoulders up and forward to palpate over each trapezius muscle surface the inferior deep cervical, accessory, and supraclavicular lymph nodes.	
Anterior midline cervical region, including hyoid bone, thyroid gland, thyroid cartilage, and larynx	• Locate the thyroid cartilage and pass the fingers up and down the thyroid gland, examining for abnormal masses and overall size. • Then place one hand on each side of the trachea and gently displace the thyroid tissue to the contralateral side of the neck for each side while the other hand manually palpates the displaced glandular tissue. • Then compare the two lobes of the gland for size and texture using visual inspection as well as manual or bimanual palpation. • Ask to swallow to check for gland mobility by visually inspecting it while it moves superiorly and then back inferiorly, possibly with a glass of water to swallow. • Finally, bidigitally palpate both the hyoid and larynx and deliberately move each one gently.	

(Continued)

Part 2: CLINICAL EXAMINATION EXERCISE: Intraoral Examination Procedure

Directions: During this exercise of an intraoral examination procedure, identify any atypical findings. Use both visual inspection and palpation during the examination, making sure to also note any atypical findings such as Fordyce spots, linea alba, exostoses, or mandibular tori. Include specific location using nearby structures such as that within the dentition. Also note any abnormal findings; if found, take nonidentifiable clinical photographs to be shared (after being granted permission) with other students and make appropriate referrals.

When examining oral mucosal surfaces, it is important to gently dry those surfaces with a gauze or air syringe so that color or texture changes will become more obvious. In addition, avoid palpation of any structures near the soft palate or pharynx to prevent the gag reflex; use only visual inspection in this area.

Regions	Steps	Findings
Oral cavity, including lips, labial commissures, buccal mucosa and labial mucosa, parotid salivary glands and ducts, alveolar processes, and attached gingiva	• Visually observe the lips at rest. • Ask for a smile and then open the mouth slightly and bidigitally palpate, as well as visually inspect, the lower and upper lip in a systematic manner from one commissure to the other. • Then gently pull the lower and upper lip away from the teeth to observe the labial mucosa and then bidigitally palpate the inner lips. • Then gently pull the buccal mucosa slightly away from the teeth to bidigitally palpate the inner cheek on each side, using circular compression. • Dry the area with gauze and observe the salivary flow from each parotid duct near the parotid papillae. • Retract both the buccal mucosa and labial mucosa to visually inspect the vestibular area and gingival tissue, including the maxillary tuberosity and retromolar pad on each side. • Then digitally palpate these inner areas using circular compression.	
Palate and pharynx, including the hard and soft palates, faucial pillars, palatine tonsils, uvula, and visible parts of oropharynx and nasopharynx	• Ask to tilt the head back slightly and extend the tongue to view the palatal and pharyngeal regions while using the mouth mirror to intensify the light source. • Gently place the mouth mirror with mirror side down on the middle of the dorsal surface of the tongue and ask to say "ah." As this is done, again visually observe the soft palate with uvula as well as the visible parts of the pharynx. • Compress the hard palate with the first or second finger of one hand, avoiding circular compression as well as avoiding palpation on the soft palate so as to prevent initiating the gag reflex.	

Regions	Steps	Findings
Tongue, including all surfaces from tip to base, as well as swallowing pattern	• Ask to slightly extend the tongue and then wrap gauze around the anterior third of the tongue in order to obtain a firm grasp to visually inspect and then digitally palpate the dorsal surface. • Then turn the tongue slightly on its side to visually inspect its base and lateral borders and bidigitally palpate the lateral borders. • Ask to lift the tongue to visually inspect and digitally palpate the ventral surface. • Ask to swallow and observe the swallowing pattern while holding the lips apart, possibly with a glass of water to swallow.	
Floor of the mouth, including the submandibular and sublingual salivary glands and ducts	• Ask to lift the tongue to the palate and using the mouth mirror to intensify the light source, visually inspect the mucosa of the floor of the mouth and check the lingual frenum. • Dry each sublingual caruncle with gauze and observe the salivary flow from the ducts. • Then bimanually palpate the sublingual region by placing an index finger intraorally behind each mandibular canine, and the index finger of the opposite hand extraorally under the chin, compressing the tissue between the fingers.	

PART 1: CHAPTER WORD JUMBLES

Note: Answers can be obtained from your instructor and their Evolve Resources

Chapter 1. Introduction to Head and Neck Anatomy

1. *Name it; own it!* CMEENTRONLAU ☐☐☐☐☐☐☐☐☐☐☐☐

2. *Go to front of the class* LARNTEV ☐☐☐☐☐☐☐

3. *Split screen moment* MISLADAGITT ☐☐☐☐☐☐☐☐☐☐☐

4. *Parallel universe* LATITAGS ☐☐☐☐☐☐☐☐

5. *Pass the sliced bread* NOLOCAR ☐☐☐☐☐☐☐

6. *Morning pancake time* EVANSSRERT ☐☐☐☐☐☐☐☐☐☐

7. *Like a snowflake* NATIARIOV ☐☐☐☐☐☐☐☐☐

8. *On this side of fence* ILSITARELAP ☐☐☐☐☐☐☐☐☐☐☐

9. *Opposite views allowed* AONRTATALERCL ☐☐☐☐☐☐☐☐☐☐☐☐☐

10. *Close to the middle ground* MLIXOPAR ☐☐☐☐☐☐☐☐

Chapter 2: Surface Anatomy

1. *Between the two caterpillars* LBELALAG ☐☐☐☐☐☐☐☐

2. *Side of skull bones matey!* METAPRLO ☐☐☐☐☐☐☐☐

3. *Groovy ear piece* ASTGURTANI ☐☐☐☐☐☐☐☐☐☐

4. *Spill some sad fluid* AMRACILL ☐☐☐☐☐☐☐☐

5. *Be cheeky and fun!* CYMOGATIZ ☐☐☐☐☐☐☐☐☐

6. *Look over this joint* METPORRBUNDIMALAO ☐☐☐☐☐☐☐☐☐☐☐☐☐☐☐☐☐

7. *Grind and grow* SERMATES ☐☐☐☐☐☐☐☐

8. *Corner kissing booth* REMSISMUCO ☐☐☐☐☐☐☐☐☐☐

9. *Okay aging sign* NABLSOAIAL ☐☐☐☐☐☐☐☐☐☐

10. *Hard to reach in mouth* BUTOREYITS ☐☐☐☐☐☐☐☐☐☐

11. *Bottom back padding* MARTOORLER ☐☐☐☐☐☐☐☐☐☐

12. *Gum junction* LUGVGIACIONM ☐☐☐☐☐☐☐☐☐☐☐☐

13. *Roof of mouth tickle* AEGRU ☐☐☐☐☐
14. *Open wider!* LYARTBOMENDIRUPAG ☐☐☐☐☐☐☐☐☐☐☐☐☐☐☐
15. *Dividing the tongue top* NISMITALER ☐☐☐☐☐☐☐☐☐
16. *Fine as a thread* MOLIRIFF ☐☐☐☐☐☐☐
17. *Large mushrooms lined up* TAVLCMURALICE ☐☐☐☐☐☐☐☐☐☐☐☐
18. *Close to voice box* XYARGNAPHROYNL ☐☐☐☐☐☐☐☐☐☐☐☐
19. *Small bump on mouth floor* NERUCCLA ☐☐☐☐☐☐☐
20. *Fringe is in!* BITFRAIMA ☐☐☐☐☐☐☐☐

Chapter 3: Skeletal System

1. *Oval bony standout* CYEDOLN ☐☐☐☐☐☐☐
2. *Rough going!* YBEROSITUT ☐☐☐☐☐☐☐☐☐
3. *Elevate and celebrate* MNEENECI ☐☐☐☐☐☐☐
4. *Deeply depressed* SAFSO ☐☐☐☐☐
5. *Window in bone* REFANOM ☐☐☐☐☐☐☐
6. *Narrow peep hole* PEARUTAER ☐☐☐☐☐☐☐☐
7. *Joining together* AIRCITULANOT ☐☐☐☐☐☐☐☐☐☐☐
8. *Jagged skull lines* TESURU ☐☐☐☐☐☐
9. *Brain suitcase* CNAMIUR ☐☐☐☐☐☐☐
10. *Baby soft spot* NOLLENTAFE ☐☐☐☐☐☐☐☐☐
11. *Upside-down V-shape suture* ABMDODIALL ☐☐☐☐☐☐☐☐☐☐
12. *Superior rim to orbit* LOPRAUBRITAS ☐☐☐☐☐☐☐☐☐☐☐
13. *Nasal cavity projections* BERTINATUS ☐☐☐☐☐☐☐☐☐
14. *Plates of sphenoid* GTEDYPOIR ☐☐☐☐☐☐☐☐
15. *Mandibular nerve travel* ALOVE ☐☐☐☐☐
16. *Facial nerve tunnel* SLOYTDASTIMO ☐☐☐☐☐☐☐☐☐☐☐
17. *Largest skull opening* NAMGUM ☐☐☐☐☐☐
18. *Plated smell perforations* MRIRBOFIRC ☐☐☐☐☐☐☐☐☐
19. *Twelfth nerve skull opening* HLPGSOLOSAY ☐☐☐☐☐☐☐☐☐☐
20. *Four-sided plate* SIBALAR ☐☐☐☐☐☐☐
21. *Back midline skull bump* BRECUPERANTO ☐☐☐☐☐☐☐☐☐☐☐☐
22. *Bone deep to the temple* TLMOPRAE ☐☐☐☐☐☐
23. *Neighbor to tympanic membrane* TESMUA ☐☐☐☐☐☐
24. *Pituitary deep fossa* LYPPOHYSEAH ☐☐☐☐☐☐☐☐☐☐

25. *Trapezoidal single midline facial bone* MEVOR ☐☐☐☐☐

26. *Serves pterygopalatine ganglion* EPHETPOALANINS ☐☐☐☐☐☐☐☐☐☐☐☐☐

27. *Two articulate forming front roof* NATALIPE ☐☐☐☐☐☐☐☐

28. *Clooney chin dimple fused in childhood* SSMHYPSIY ☐☐☐☐☐☐☐☐☐

29. *Notch between process and condyle* RANBILUDAM ☐☐☐☐☐☐☐☐☐☐

30. *First with skull articulation* STAAL ☐☐☐☐☐

Chapter 4: Muscular System

1. *Largest cervical* DTERMADLEOCINOSTOIS ☐☐☐☐☐☐☐☐☐☐☐☐☐☐☐☐☐☐☐

2. *Muscle shrugged* PRESAZIUT ☐☐☐☐☐☐☐☐☐

3. *Scalp movement* CLIERAPIAN ☐☐☐☐☐☐☐☐☐☐

4. *Lip point of muscle contact* SOLOIDUM ☐☐☐☐☐☐☐☐

5. *Gives faux smile* TYSOUAZICMG ☐☐☐☐☐☐☐☐☐☐☐

6. *Narrows mandibular vestibule* TENSMALI ☐☐☐☐☐☐☐☐

7. *Neck bands with age* MLATSPAY ☐☐☐☐☐☐☐☐

8. *Muscles to chew on* NASTITACIOM ☐☐☐☐☐☐☐☐☐☐☐

9. *Parallels nearby medial pterygoid* TASEMERS ☐☐☐☐☐☐☐☐

10. *Deepest chew muscle* LIDEAM ☐☐☐☐☐☐

11. *Fan-shaped within its own fossa* PEMSTOIRAL ☐☐☐☐☐☐☐☐☐☐

12. *Muscles superior to hyoid* HUDRASYOIP ☐☐☐☐☐☐☐☐☐☐

13. *Has two slips to elevate hyoid* OTDLSYOIHY ☐☐☐☐☐☐☐☐☐☐

14. *Muscles inferior to hyoid* IDHROFYAIN ☐☐☐☐☐☐☐☐☐☐

15. *Two bellies form anterior cervical triangle* CAGISTRID ☐☐☐☐☐☐☐☐☐

16. *Between to mandibular rami* MDLIHYOOY ☐☐☐☐☐☐☐☐☐

17. *At genial tubercles onward to hyoid* DYNIOOHIGE ☐☐☐☐☐☐☐☐☐☐

18. *Two bellies that depress hyoid* DOOMHYIO ☐☐☐☐☐☐☐☐

19. *Off sternum near clavicle* SYTEDNOHOIR ☐☐☐☐☐☐☐☐☐☐☐

20. *All end with glossus tag* ECNSITRIX ☐☐☐☐☐☐☐☐☐

21. *Fan-shaped largest tongue muscle* SENIUSLOSGOG ☐☐☐☐☐☐☐☐☐☐☐☐

22. *Lateral/posterior pharyngeal walls* SCONTTRICORS ☐☐☐☐☐☐☐☐☐☐☐☐

23. *Anterior faucial pillar* PALGSTAOOLSSU ☐☐☐☐☐☐☐☐☐☐☐☐☐

24. *Posterior faucial pillar* GALHSYPAARONPEUT ☐☐☐☐☐☐☐☐☐☐☐☐☐☐☐☐

25. *Entirely within hanging throat tissue* AUVLU ☐☐☐☐☐

Chapter 5: Temporomandibular Joint

1. *Oval-shaped TMJ depression* SAFSO ☐☐☐☐☐
2. *Sharper ridge* POGTSLONEID ☐☐☐☐☐☐☐☐☐☐
3. *Facial bone with TMJ* BENDIMLA ☐☐☐☐☐☐☐☐
4. *Cranial bone with TMJ* ROMPETAL ☐☐☐☐☐☐☐☐
5. *Wraps around TMJ completely* EAPLUSC ☐☐☐☐☐☐☐
6. *Two cavities dividing TMJ* VLNOSIAY ☐☐☐☐☐☐☐☐
7. *Synovial lubrication* DLUIF ☐☐☐☐☐
8. *Mandible joined to cranium* GLIMAESNT ☐☐☐☐☐☐☐☐☐
9. *Capsule ligament thickening* REMPARIBANDOMULOT ☐☐☐☐☐☐☐☐☐☐☐☐☐☐☐☐☐
10. *Cervical fascia ligament thickening* BTYLUNAMDISOLAR ☐☐☐☐☐☐☐☐☐☐☐☐☐☐☐
11. *Mandibular foramen overlap* SLHUNONAMDIBEPAR ☐☐☐☐☐☐☐☐☐☐☐☐☐☐☐☐
12. *TMJ forward/backward disc movement* LGINIDG ☐☐☐☐☐☐☐
13. *Lowering of lower jaw* SESPRENIOD ☐☐☐☐☐☐☐☐☐☐
14. *Raising of lower jaw* VLEEOTIAN ☐☐☐☐☐☐☐☐☐
15. *Lower jaw backward* NECRATTIOR ☐☐☐☐☐☐☐☐☐☐
16. *Lower jaw forward* PNUTROSIOR ☐☐☐☐☐☐☐☐☐☐
17. *Shifting lower jaw to side* DEOVINTIA ☐☐☐☐☐☐☐☐☐
18. *Resting mandible* LEANARCCE ☐☐☐☐☐☐☐☐☐
19. *Pathology with TMJ* RIRODDES ☐☐☐☐☐☐☐☐
20. *Dislocation of both jaws* BASLUXUTOIN ☐☐☐☐☐☐☐☐☐☐☐

Chapter 6: Vascular system

1. *Texting blood vessels* ATNSAIMOSOS ☐☐☐☐☐☐☐☐☐☐☐
2. *Network group* XLESUP ☐☐☐☐☐☐
3. *Middle smooth layer* EIAMD ☐☐☐☐☐
4. *From heart carrying blood away* YATRER ☐☐☐☐☐☐
5. *Smaller-diameter arteriole* CPYILLARA ☐☐☐☐☐☐☐☐☐
6. *Smaller-diameter vein* ENLUVE ☐☐☐☐☐☐
7. *Blood-filled venous spaces* NIESUSS ☐☐☐☐☐☐☐
8. *Left side big artery* TAOAR ☐☐☐☐☐
9. *Branchless carotid within own sheath* MOOCMN ☐☐☐☐☐☐

10. *Lateral to common carotid* LABCSAVIUN ⬚⬚⬚⬚⬚⬚⬚⬚⬚⬚

11. *Supplies eye and orbit* IPHTMALHOC ⬚⬚⬚⬚⬚⬚⬚⬚⬚⬚

12. *Artery without its named nerve* AINGULL ⬚⬚⬚⬚⬚⬚⬚

13. *Supplies mylohyoid* SBULLGINAU ⬚⬚⬚⬚⬚⬚⬚⬚⬚⬚

14. *Artery with complicated path* LACIAF ⬚⬚⬚⬚⬚⬚

15. *Terminal branch of facial artery* GNAALUR ⬚⬚⬚⬚⬚⬚⬚

16. *Largest external carotid terminal* LAXILMAYR ⬚⬚⬚⬚⬚⬚⬚⬚⬚

17. *Exits mandibular canal via mental foramen* LETNAM ⬚⬚⬚⬚⬚⬚

18. *Supply mandibular anteriors* CINIVISE ⬚⬚⬚⬚⬚⬚⬚⬚

19. *Supplies buccinator* BCULCA ⬚⬚⬚⬚⬚⬚

20. *Drains into internal jugular vein* LIAFAC ⬚⬚⬚⬚⬚⬚

21. *Lingual vein for tongue top* RODLSA ⬚⬚⬚⬚⬚⬚

22. *Drains floor of mouth* SUANBILGUL ⬚⬚⬚⬚⬚⬚⬚⬚⬚⬚

23. *Forms external jugular vein* REMRANTADIRULOB ⬚⬚⬚⬚⬚⬚⬚⬚⬚⬚⬚⬚⬚⬚⬚

24. *Plexus surrounding maxillary artery* PDEGRYOIT ⬚⬚⬚⬚⬚⬚⬚⬚⬚

25. *Drains most of head and neck structures* RULGUAJ ⬚⬚⬚⬚⬚⬚⬚

Chapter 7: Glandular Tissue

1. *Gland with duct* XEOCINRE ⬚⬚⬚⬚⬚⬚⬚⬚

2. *Gland without duct* CONDRIENE ⬚⬚⬚⬚⬚⬚⬚⬚⬚

3. *Secrete tears* LIARMALC ⬚⬚⬚⬚⬚⬚⬚⬚

4. *Tear duct* MASOLCLARINA ⬚⬚⬚⬚⬚⬚⬚⬚⬚⬚⬚⬚

5. *Production by salivary glands* SIVLAA ⬚⬚⬚⬚⬚⬚

6. *The top three* OARMJ ⬚⬚⬚⬚⬚

7. *Largest spit maker* PAIRDTO ⬚⬚⬚⬚⬚⬚⬚

8. *Other parotid duct name* NNETSES ⬚⬚⬚⬚⬚⬚⬚

9. *Enlarged tender parotid* SUPMM ⬚⬚⬚⬚⬚

10. *Parotid enlargement* PASRTTOII ⬚⬚⬚⬚⬚⬚⬚⬚⬚

11. *Second-largest spit maker* NUMASDIBULABR ⬚⬚⬚⬚⬚⬚⬚⬚⬚⬚⬚⬚⬚

12. *Other submandibular duct name* HORTAWN ⬚⬚⬚⬚⬚⬚⬚

13. *Smallest major spit maker* BUSLUGNIAL ⬚⬚⬚⬚⬚⬚⬚⬚⬚⬚

14. *Collective of sublingual ducts* IVUINRS ⬚⬚⬚⬚⬚⬚⬚

15. *Other name of sublingual duct* HORTBALIN ⬚⬚⬚⬚⬚⬚⬚⬚⬚

16. *Special minor spit maker* BENRE ☐☐☐☐☐

17. *Reduced spit production* SHPYALVIATIOON ☐☐☐☐☐☐☐☐☐☐☐☐

18. *Fancy name for dry mouth* XMERISTOOA ☐☐☐☐☐☐☐☐☐

19. *Gland products stimulating times* TRYHODI ☐☐☐☐☐☐☐

20. *Adjacent or within thyroid* PHYADATROIR ☐☐☐☐☐☐☐☐☐☐

Chapter 8: Nervous System

1. *Superior alveolar may not home* MEDIDL ☐☐☐☐☐☐

2. *Overlapping terminal nerve fibers* CRORSOVES ☐☐☐☐☐☐☐☐☐

3. *Cutaneous upper lip branches merger* BINTRAORIFAL ☐☐☐☐☐☐☐☐☐☐☐

4. *Through foramen rotundum* RAILLAMXY ☐☐☐☐☐☐☐☐☐

5. *First division of fifth* COPHTHALIM ☐☐☐☐☐☐☐☐☐☐

6. *Bulge in petrous part* TMEGIRINAL ☐☐☐☐☐☐☐☐☐☐

7. *What happens in organs stays in organs* AGUSV ☐☐☐☐☐

8. *Innervates parotid gland* LGOPSOHALYNGESAR ☐☐☐☐☐☐☐☐☐☐☐☐☐☐☐☐

9. *Makes muscles of expression work* CFIAAL ☐☐☐☐☐☐

10. *Serves anterior hard palate* NANPOESALATI ☐☐☐☐☐☐☐☐☐☐☐

11. *Palatine nerve keeping tonsils happy* SLEESR ☐☐☐☐☐☐

12. *Superior alveolar maxillary sinus coverage* PROSERIOT ☐☐☐☐☐☐☐☐☐

13. *Innervates lower lip* ANTELM ☐☐☐☐☐☐☐

14. *Bifid alveolar with double mandibular canal* FONIRIER ☐☐☐☐☐☐☐☐

15. *Lingual nerve ganglion communication* SMUBRALNDIBUA ☐☐☐☐☐☐☐☐☐☐☐☐☐

16. *Associated with inferior dental plexus* VINSCIIE ☐☐☐☐☐☐☐☐

17. *May serve mandibular first molar* MDOHYYOIL ☐☐☐☐☐☐☐☐☐

18. *Neuralgia with trigger zones* ATRIILMGEN ☐☐☐☐☐☐☐☐☐☐

19. *BFFs with chorda tympani nerve* FAACLI ☐☐☐☐☐☐

20. *Facial paralysis type with gland injection* TTASIENNR ☐☐☐☐☐☐☐☐☐

21. *Miswiring of nerves* SNNIYKIESS ☐☐☐☐☐☐☐☐☐☐

22. *Crock tears with lunch* LYCERHAPRIMNTIOA ☐☐☐☐☐☐☐☐☐☐☐☐☐☐☐☐

23. *Half of Bell palsy* TIONFECIN ☐☐☐☐☐☐☐☐☐

24. *Facial expression muscles after stroke* PLAYIRASS ☐☐☐☐☐☐☐☐☐

25. *Riding with inferior alveolar* GILLUAN ☐☐☐☐☐☐☐

Chapter 9: Anatomy of Local Anesthesia

1. *Involved single skull bone* MEBNDIAL ☐☐☐☐☐☐☐☐

2. *Injection for small area* ROPSATERIUSPEAL ☐☐☐☐☐☐☐☐☐☐☐☐☐

3. *Injection for larger area* KLOCB ☐☐☐☐☐

4. *Never inject with this present* SACBSES ☐☐☐☐☐☐☐

5. *Dental arch with way better anesthesia* YALXILARM ☐☐☐☐☐☐☐☐☐

6. *Superior alveolar not always accounted for* DIEDMIL ☐☐☐☐☐☐

7. *Surface of maxilla for PSA block* LINFRAAMETPOR ☐☐☐☐☐☐☐☐☐☐☐☐

8. *Extraoral lesion with too deep PSA block* MEAHOTAM ☐☐☐☐☐☐☐☐

9. *Landmark for ASA block* ANENIC ☐☐☐☐☐☐

10. *Anesthetizes ASA and MSA nerves* AOTINFRARBIL ☐☐☐☐☐☐☐☐☐☐☐

11. *Foramen inferior to lower orbit rim* LIONTFRARBIA ☐☐☐☐☐☐☐☐☐☐☐

12. *Palatine block maxillary posterior sextant* GRETARE ☐☐☐☐☐☐☐

13. *Palatine block maxillary anterior sextant* ENAINPSOLAAT ☐☐☐☐☐☐☐☐☐☐☐

14. *Landmark for NP block* PLAAPIL ☐☐☐☐☐☐☐

15. *Dental arch with most variation* MIBNDALE ☐☐☐☐☐☐☐☐

16. *Alveolar block used most commonly* FIONRERI ☐☐☐☐☐☐☐☐

17. *Bundles anesthetized on posterior mandible* METLAN ☐☐☐☐☐☐

18. *Block given with IA block* CBULCA ☐☐☐☐☐☐

19. *Double trouble mandibular foramen* FIBID ☐☐☐☐☐

20. *Mandibular landmark for IA block* MARUS ☐☐☐☐☐

21. *Nerve that gets shocked!* ALIGNUL ☐☐☐☐☐☐☐

22. *Abnormal sensation in area* SPAERSTHEIA ☐☐☐☐☐☐☐☐☐☐

23. *Padded landmark buccal block* MREOTROALR ☐☐☐☐☐☐☐☐☐☐

24. *Tooth nearby mental block* PRERLOMA ☐☐☐☐☐☐☐☐

25. *Block also uses mental foramen landmark* IENCISVI ☐☐☐☐☐☐☐☐

26. *Gow-Gates covers this nerve for sure!* MHYDOIYOL ☐☐☐☐☐☐☐☐☐

27. *Notch for Gow-Gates block* RINCERTAGIT ☐☐☐☐☐☐☐☐☐☐

28. *V-A mandibular block okay with this!* MRUSTIS ☐☐☐☐☐☐☐

29. *Mucosa needle enters with V-A mandibular block* BLUCAC ☐☐☐☐☐

30. *Decreased with V-A mandibular block* NASIRATIOP ☐☐☐☐☐☐☐☐☐☐

Chapter 10: Lymphatic System

1. *System of channels* SESEVLS ☐☐☐☐☐☐☐
2. *Fluid in said channels* PLMYH ☐☐☐☐☐
3. *Bean-shaped lymphatic groupies* DONSE ☐☐☐☐☐
4. *Arrives into the node* NAFEREFT ☐☐☐☐☐☐☐☐
5. *Exits the node* TREFFEEN ☐☐☐☐☐☐☐☐
6. *Drains first* MRYPARI ☐☐☐☐☐☐☐
7. *Drains next* DOCENSRAY ☐☐☐☐☐☐☐☐☐
8. *Masses of oral cavity lymphoid tissue* STINSOL ☐☐☐☐☐☐☐
9. *Lymphatic vessels converge* DTCUS ☐☐☐☐☐
10. *Right side converge to trunk* RULUGAJ ☐☐☐☐☐☐☐
11. *Left side converge to duct* TCIORAHC ☐☐☐☐☐☐☐☐
12. *Nodes at posterior base of head* COACPIITL ☐☐☐☐☐☐☐☐☐
13. *Nodes zig-zagging across face* CLAFIA ☐☐☐☐☐☐
14. *Nodes at level of atlas* LEGRPOHAYNTREAR ☐☐☐☐☐☐☐☐☐☐☐☐☐☐☐
15. *Nodes also known by Roman numerals* CLEVRICA ☐☐☐☐☐☐☐☐
16. *Feeling nodes under chin* TUABMENSL ☐☐☐☐☐☐☐☐☐
17. *Juglar nodes near external jugular vein* LETERNAX ☐☐☐☐☐☐☐☐
18. *Tonsillar node feeling large!* CUDGULGOIASTRIJ ☐☐☐☐☐☐☐☐☐☐☐☐☐☐☐
19. *Nodes draining lateral cervical triangles* SUAPRCARLAVICUL ☐☐☐☐☐☐☐☐☐☐☐☐☐☐☐
20. *Tonsils between the pillars* ALPATIEN ☐☐☐☐☐☐☐☐
21. *Enlarge tonsils/nodes* PHYLMPADONEATHY ☐☐☐☐☐☐☐☐☐☐☐☐☐☐☐
22. *Nodal inflammation* LIYSPHAEDNITM ☐☐☐☐☐☐☐☐☐☐☐☐☐
23. *Traveling neoplasm* MEISTASTAS ☐☐☐☐☐☐☐☐☐☐
24. *Cancer by way of blood vessels* MARNCIOCA ☐☐☐☐☐☐☐☐☐
25. *Dental professional's cancer weapon* TALNAPIOP ☐☐☐☐☐☐☐☐☐

Chapter 11: Fasciae and Spaces

1. *Layers upon layers* SFAACI ☐☐☐☐☐☐
2. *Fascial planes* SESPAC ☐☐☐☐☐☐
3. *Fascia encloses expression muscles* SFIUPEARCIL ☐☐☐☐☐☐☐☐☐☐☐
4. *Fascia with medial pterygoid muscle* TERDYGOIP ☐☐☐☐☐☐☐☐☐

5. *Most external layer of deep cervical fascia* VISGNETIN ⬚⬚⬚⬚⬚⬚⬚⬚⬚

6. *Bilateral tube with lots of structures!* CDARIOT ⬚⬚⬚⬚⬚⬚⬚

7. *Parallel to carotid sheath* VILSCEAR ⬚⬚⬚⬚⬚⬚⬚

8. *Deepest layer of deep cervical fascia* BARTEVREL ⬚⬚⬚⬚⬚⬚⬚⬚⬚

9. *Space located medial to buccinator* RESTIUBLAV ⬚⬚⬚⬚⬚⬚⬚⬚⬚⬚

10. *Floor of space is canine fossa* CENINA ⬚⬚⬚⬚⬚⬚

11. *Space between buccinator and masseter* CABCUL ⬚⬚⬚⬚⬚⬚

12. *Space with much of facial nerve* APRDTIO ⬚⬚⬚⬚⬚⬚⬚

13. *Space with entire mandible* TASICATOMR ⬚⬚⬚⬚⬚⬚⬚⬚

14. *Swelling space limited by temporalis fascia* TPAMEORL ⬚⬚⬚⬚⬚⬚⬚⬚

15. *IA nerve space* RTEYGRMOANIDBULAP ⬚⬚⬚⬚⬚⬚⬚⬚⬚⬚⬚⬚⬚⬚⬚⬚⬚

16. *Spaces within neck that communicate!* CEIVARCL ⬚⬚⬚⬚⬚⬚⬚⬚

17. *Danger neck space* LETROHPANYRGEAR ⬚⬚⬚⬚⬚⬚⬚⬚⬚⬚⬚⬚⬚⬚⬚

18. *Compartment containing spinal cord* LVEBTERRA ⬚⬚⬚⬚⬚⬚⬚⬚⬚

19. *Compartment containing thyroid* VILCSERA ⬚⬚⬚⬚⬚⬚⬚⬚

20. *Compartment with carotid sheath* SAUAVCLR ⬚⬚⬚⬚⬚⬚⬚⬚

Chapter 12: Spread of Infection

1. *Balancing residing bugs* MIABCROOIT ⬚⬚⬚⬚⬚⬚⬚⬚⬚⬚

2. *Bad bugs* GAHTOPENS ⬚⬚⬚⬚⬚⬚⬚⬚⬚

3. *Multiplication and invasion: oh my!* NIICFETON ⬚⬚⬚⬚⬚⬚⬚⬚⬚

4. *Dental infection by oral pathogens* CODONITOGEN ⬚⬚⬚⬚⬚⬚⬚⬚⬚⬚⬚

5. *Reason for increased dental infection risk* MIOLFIB ⬚⬚⬚⬚⬚⬚⬚

6. *Localized entrapment of pathogens* SASBSCE ⬚⬚⬚⬚⬚⬚⬚

7. *Icky substance with fluctuance* SPUTUPRAION ⬚⬚⬚⬚⬚⬚⬚⬚⬚⬚⬚

8. *Tract that forms* FSIAUL ⬚⬚⬚⬚⬚⬚

9. *Fistula opening* ATOSM ⬚⬚⬚⬚⬚

10. *Elevated lesion with suppuration* PUESUTL ⬚⬚⬚⬚⬚⬚⬚

11. *Diffuse inflammation of soft tissue spaces* TLCELULIIS ⬚⬚⬚⬚⬚⬚⬚⬚⬚⬚

12. *Inflammation of bone marrow* OMEYISTOELITS ⬚⬚⬚⬚⬚⬚⬚⬚⬚⬚⬚⬚⬚

13. *Piece of dead bone surrounding exudate* QUEESUTRMS ⬚⬚⬚⬚⬚⬚⬚⬚⬚⬚

14. *New bone forming near sequestrum* INCLVOURM ⬚⬚⬚⬚⬚⬚⬚⬚⬚

15. *Infections taking advantage* OPUOCPRTNISTI ⬚⬚⬚⬚⬚⬚⬚⬚⬚⬚⬚⬚

16. *Bacteria within vascular system* CABMTEREIA ⬚⬚⬚⬚⬚⬚⬚⬚⬚⬚

17. *Transport infected into venous sinus* HROOMTBSIS ⬚⬚⬚⬚⬚⬚⬚⬚⬚

18. *Eye nerve with cavernous sinus thrombosis* ABCDENSU ⬚⬚⬚⬚⬚⬚⬚

19. *Infection of brain part* MNEINTIGIS ⬚⬚⬚⬚⬚⬚⬚⬚⬚⬚

20. *Cellulitis of submandibular space* NAGNIA ⬚⬚⬚⬚⬚⬚

PART 2: CHAPTER CROSSWORD PUZZLES

Note: Answers can be obtained from your instructor and their Evolve Resources

CHAPTER 1: INTRODUCTION TO THE HEAD AND NECK ANATOMY

Crossword Puzzle 1

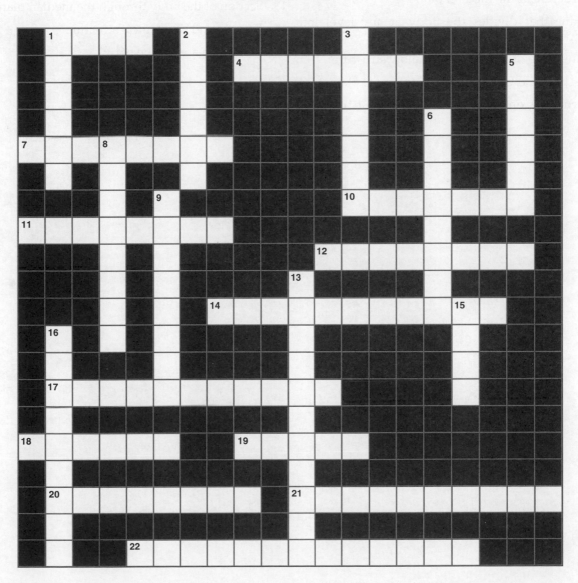

Across

1. Structure located inward away from the body surface.
4. Part directed toward anterior.
7. Any plane of the body parallel to the median plane.
10. Area that is farther away from the midsagittal plane of the body or structure.
11. Outer side of the wall of a hollow structure.
12. Area closer to the median plane of the body.
14. Structures on the same side of the body.
17. Structures located toward the surface of the body.
18. Structure at the median plane.
19. Plane that divides the body at any level into superior and inferior parts.
20. Inner side of the wall of a hollow structure.
21. Section of the body through any axial plane.
22. Structures on the opposite side of the body.

Down

1. Area that is farther away from the median plane of the body.
2. Area that is closer to the midsagittal plane of the body or structure.
3. Plane that divides the body at any level into anterior and posterior parts.
5. Part that is directed toward the posterior.
6. Area that faces toward the head of the body and away from the feet.
8. Area that faces away from the head and towards the feet of the body.
9. Front area of a body.
13. Section of the body through the median plane.
15. Pointed end of a conical structure.
16. Back of an area of the body.

CHAPTER 2: SURFACE ANATOMY

Crossword Puzzle 2

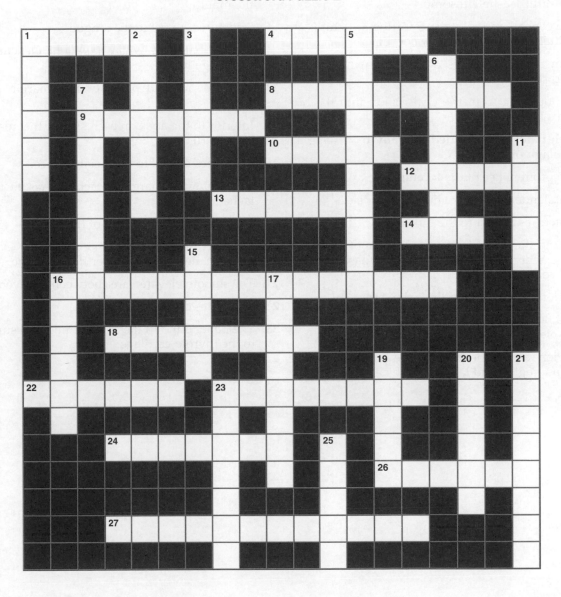

Across

1. Layers of soft tissue overlying the bones of the braincase.
4. Facial structures closest to the inner cheek.
8. Zone where each lip has a darker reddish appearance than surrounding skin.
9. The oval flap of the ear that reminds one of a beautiful seashell in some.
10. The eyeball and all its supporting structures are contained within the bony socket.
12. Firm irregular ridges of tissue on the anterior hard palate.
13. The opening from the oral region into the oropharynx.
14. Each nares are bounded laterally by a winglike cartilaginous structure.
16. The prominence of the forehead.
18. The slender threadlike lingual papillae.
22. Structures closest to the lips.
23. On the skin superior to the midline of the upper lip, extending downward from the nasal septum, is a vertical groove.
24 Underlying the upper lip is the upper jaw.
26 The fleshy protuberance of the earlobe that can get pierced.
27 Region of the head is located inferior to the orbital region and lateral to the nasal region.

Down

1. On the eyeball, this is the white area.
2. The oral cavity also provides the entrance into this muscular tube.
3. The inner surface of the marginal gingiva faces a space.
5. The upper and lower lips meet at each corner of the mouth.
6. Structures closest to the tongue.
7. Muscle palpated when a patient clenches the teeth together.
11. The superior and posterior free margin of the auricle.
15. Inferior to the apex on each side of the nose that is a nostril.
16. Structures closest to the facial surface.
17. At the gingival margin of each tooth is the nonattached gingiva.
19. The opening in the center of the iris.
20. The part of the auricle anterior to the external acoustic meatus is a smaller flap of tissue.
21. The smooth elevated area between the eyebrows.
23. Structures closest to the palate.
25. The bone found in the anterior midline, superior to the thyroid cartilage.

CHAPTER 3: SKELETAL SYSTEM

Crossword Puzzle 3

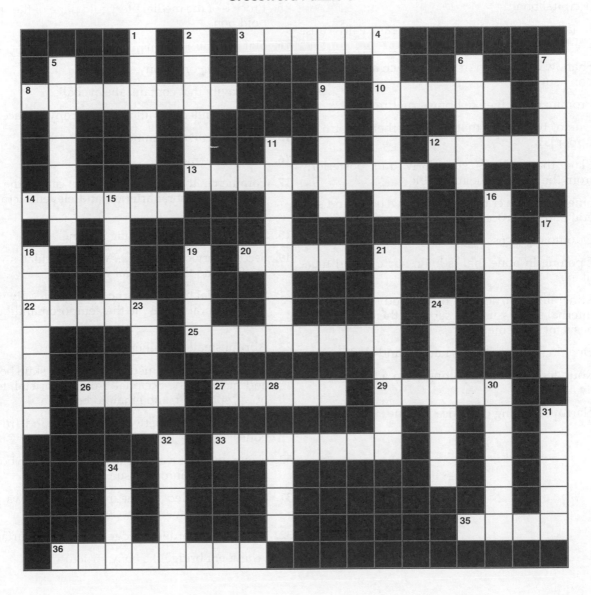

Across

3. Small opening in bone.

8. Paired facial bones that help form the anterior medial corner of the orbit.

10. Structure composed of both the cranial bones or cranium and facial bones.

12. First cervical vertebra, which articulates with the occipital bone.

13. Inflammation of the sinus that can really cause pain!

14. Shallow depression or groove such as that on the bony surface.

20. Prominent bridgelike bony structure

21. One of two bones that fuse together to form the upper jaw.

22. Plate that extends superiorly and posteriorly from the body of the mandible.

25. Single midline cranial bone with a body and several pairs of processes.

26. Odontoid process of the second cervical vertebra.

27. Opening in bone that is long, narrow, and tube-like.

29. Mineralized structures of the body that protect internal soft tissue and serve as the biomechanic basis for movement.

33 Opening in bone that is narrow and cleftlike.

35 Rounded surface projecting from a bony surface by a neck.

36 Narrow opening or orifice in bone.

Down

1. Site of a junction or union between two or more bones.

2. Opening or canal in the bone.

4. Area on the petrous part of the temporal bone that contains the air cells and on which the large cervical muscles attach.

5. Process of the medial pterygoid plate of the sphenoid bone.

6. Flat structure of bone.

7. Depression on a bony surface.

9. Eye cavity that contains the eyeball.

11. Small rounded elevation on the bony surface.

15. Small hornlike prominence.

16. Roof of the mouth.

17. Foramen in the occipital bone that carries the spinal cord, vertebral arteries, and eleventh cranial nerve.

18. Short windowlike opening in bone.

19. Second cervical vertebra, which articulates with the first and third cervical vertebrae.

21. Single facial bone that articulates bilaterally with the temporal bones at the temporomandibular joints.

23. Abrupt small prominence of bone.

24. Structure that is formed by the cranial skull bones and includes the occipital, frontal, parietal, temporal, sphenoid, and ethmoid bones.

28. Midline junction between the nasal and frontal bones.

30. Generally immovable articulation in which bones are joined by fibrous tissue.

31. Bone suspended in the neck that allows the attachment of many muscles.

32. Roughened border or ridge on the bone surface.

34. Prominent bridgelike bony structure.

CHAPTER 4: MUSCULAR SYSTEM

Crossword Puzzle 4

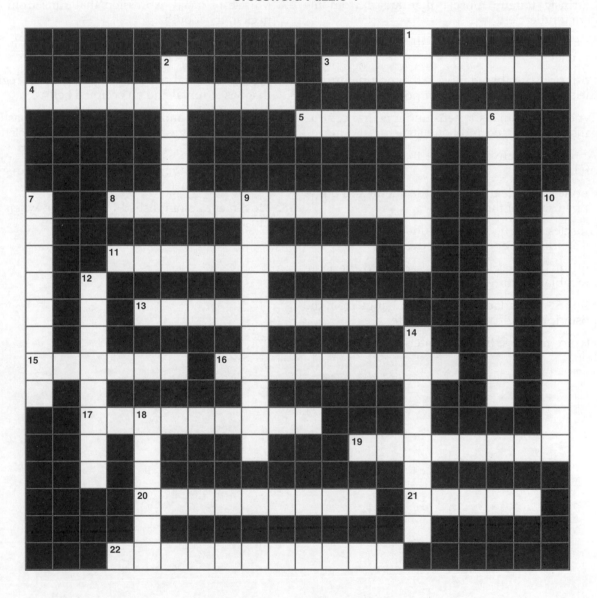

Across

3. Suprahyoid muscle with an anterior and a posterior belly.

4. Muscle of mastication that fills the temporal fossa.

5. Muscle of facial expression in the mouth region that raises the chin.

8. Extrinsic tongue muscle that arises from the genial tubercles.

11. Muscle of facial expression that forms a part of the cheek.

13. Posterior suprahyoid muscle that originates from the styloid process of the temporal bone.

15. Type of tissue that shortens under neural control, causing soft tissue and bony structures to move.

16. Anterior suprahyoid muscle that forms the floor of the mouth.

17. Cervical muscle that covers the lateral and posterior surfaces of the neck.

19. Muscles of the neck that include the sternocleidomastoid and trapezius muscles.

20. End of the muscle that is attached to the more movable structure.

21. Midline muscular structure that hangs from the posterior margin of the soft palate.

22. Hyoid muscles that are inferior to the hyoid bone.

Down

1. Loss of action of the muscles.

2. End of the muscle that is attached to the least movable structure.

6. Hyoid muscles located superior to the hyoid bone that can be further divided by their anterior or posterior relationship to the hyoid bone.

7. Muscle of facial expression that runs from the neck to the mouth.

9. Anterior suprahyoid muscle that is deep to the mylohyoid muscle.

10. Muscle of facial expression in the scalp region that has a frontal and an occipital belly.

12. Most obvious and strongest muscle of mastication that enlarges through grinding and clenching.

14. Muscle of facial expression in the mouth region that is used when smiling widely.

18. Movement accomplished by a muscle when the muscle fibers contract.

CHAPTER 5: TEMPOROMANDIBULAR JOINT

Crossword Puzzle 5

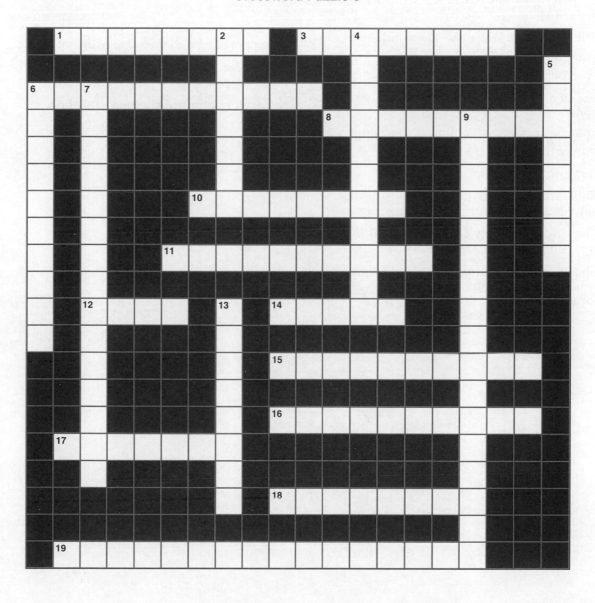

Across

1. This landmark is positioned anterior to the articular fossa and consists of a smooth rounded ridge.

3. Can involve one or both temporomandibular joints.

6. Posterior to the articular fossa is a sharper ridge.

8. Raising of the lower jaw.

10. Cranial bone that articulates with the mandible at the TMJ.

11. Bringing of the lower jaw backward.

12. This can, as a person ages, become thinner or even perforated.

14. Site of a junction or union between two or more bones.

15. The TMJ is innervated by the mandibular division of this nerve.

16. Lowering of the lower jaw.

17. This wraps around the margin of the articular eminence and articular fossa superiorly.

18. The disc completely divides the TMJ into these two compartments or spaces.

19. This ligament runs from the angular spine of the sphenoid bone to the lingula of the mandibular foramen.

Down

2. Projection of bone from the mandibular ramus that participates in the temporomandibular joint.

4. Acute episode of temporomandibular joint disorder in which both joints become dislocated often due to excessive mandibular protrusion and depression.

5. Facial bone that articulates with the temporal bone at the head of the mandibular condyle.

6. Bringing of the lower jaw forward.

7. This ligament runs from the styloid process of the temporal bone to the angle of the mandible.

9. This ligament prevents the excessive retraction or moving backward of the mandible.

13. Band of fibrous tissue connecting bones.

CHAPTER 6: VASCULAR SYSTEM

Crossword Puzzle 6

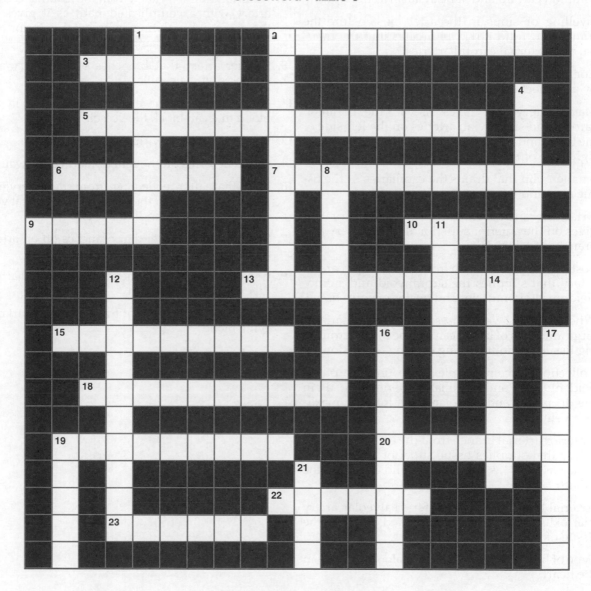

Across

2. Vein from the arm that drains the external jugular vein and then joins with the internal jugular vein to form the brachiocephalic vein.

3. Network of blood vessels, usually veins.

5. Artery that branches directly off the aorta on the right side of the body and gives rise to the right common carotid and subclavian arteries.

6. Swelling or sinus in the artery just before the common carotid artery bifurcates into the internal and external carotid arteries.

7. Communication of a blood vessel with another by a connecting channel.

9. Major artery that gives rise to the common carotid and subclavian arteries on the left side of the body and to the brachiocephalic artery on the right side of the body.

10. Smaller vein that drains the capillaries of the tissue area and then joins larger veins.

13. Arterial branch from the maxillary artery that gives off the anterior superior alveolar artery and branches to the orbit.

15. Posterior arterial branch from the external carotid artery that supplies the suprahyoid and sternocleidomastoid muscles and posterior scalp tissue.

18. When a blood vessel is seriously traumatized, large amounts of blood can escape into surrounding tissue without clotting causing this lesion.

19. Collection of veins or plexus around the pterygoid muscles and maxillary arteries that drain the deep face and alveolar veins into the maxillary vein.

20. Anterior arterial branch from the external carotid artery that supplies tissue superior to the hyoid bone, as well as the tongue and floor of the mouth.

22. Arterial branch from the inferior alveolar artery that exits the mental foramen and supplies the tissue of the chin.

23. Type of blood vessel that carries blood away from the heart.

Down

1. Bruise that results when a blood vessel is injured and a small amount of blood escapes into the surrounding tissue and clots.

2. Vein from the arm that drains the external jugular vein and then joins with the internal jugular vein to form the brachiocephalic vein.

4. Anterior arterial branch from the external carotid artery with a complicated path as it gives off the ascending palatine, submental, inferior and superior labial, and angular arteries.

8. Smaller artery that branches off an artery and connects with a capillary.

11. Foreign material or thrombus traveling in the blood that can block the vessel.

12. Bacteria traveling within the blood system.

14. Clot that forms on the inner blood vessel wall.

16. Vein that after collecting from the pterygoid plexus merges with the superficial temporal vein to form the retromandibular vein.

17. Smaller blood vessel that branches off an arteriole to supply blood directly to tissue.

19. Can be palpated from the common carotid artery given the right situation.

21. Type of blood vessel that travels to the heart carrying blood.

CHAPTER 7: GLANDULAR TISSUE

Crossword Puzzle 7

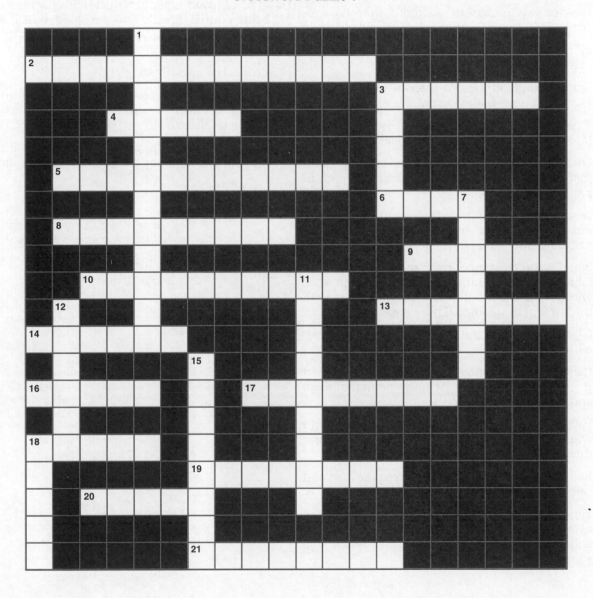

Across

2. Major gland that is located in the submandibular fossa.

3. Enlarged thyroid gland due to a disease process.

4. Sublingual gland located in this structure.

5. Small endocrine glands located close to or even inside the thyroid gland.

6. Passageway to carry the secretion from the exocrine gland to the location where it will be used.

8. Hormone produced and secreted by the thyroid gland directly into the blood.

9. Endocrine gland located inferior to the thyroid gland and deep to the sternum.

10. T-cell type that matures in the gland in response to stimulation by thymus hormones.

13. Duct associated with the parotid salivary gland that opens into the oral cavity at the parotid papilla.

14. Lesion that has dye run through it to show the blockage of saliva in a major salivary gland resulting from stone formation.

16. Small glands scattered in the tissue of the buccal, labial, and lingual mucosa, soft and hard palates, and floor of the mouth, which is associated with the circumvallate lingual papillae.

17. Gland in a fossa of the frontal bone that produces a fluid or tears.

18. Large paired glands with associated named ducts that include the parotid, submandibular, and sublingual glands.

19. Papilla near the midline of the floor of the mouth where both the sublingual and submandibular ducts open into the oral cavity.

20. Blocking the drainage of saliva from the duct and causing gland enlargement and tenderness.

21. Type of gland with an associated duct that serves as a passageway for the secretion so it can be emptied directly into the location where the secretion is to be used.

Down

1. The lacrimal fluid ends up in this structure after passing over the eyeball.

3. Structure that produces a chemical secretion necessary for body functioning.

7. Endocrine gland having two lobes and located inferior to the thyroid cartilage.

11. Type of gland without a duct, with the secretion being poured directly into the blood, which then carries the secretion to the region in which it is to be used.

12. Product of the salivary glands.

15. Lesion in a minor salivary gland due to severance of the duct from trauma and then blockage of saliva.

18. Viral infection of the parotid salivary gland that is being prevented by a childhood vaccination.

CHAPTER 8: NERVOUS SYSTEM

Crossword Puzzle 8

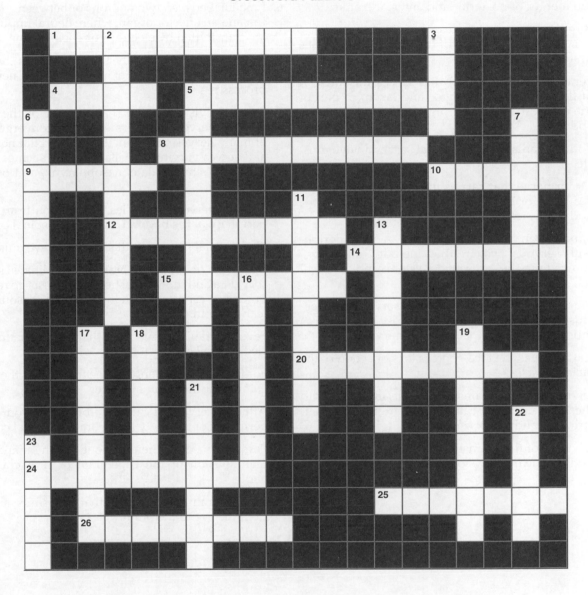

Across

1. Our nerve, the dental nerve!

4. Division of the brainstem that connects the medulla with the cerebellum.

5. Third cranial nerve (III) that serves some of the eye muscles.

8. Division of the trigeminal nerve that is formed by the merger of posterior and anterior trunks.

9. Bundle of neural processes outside the central nervous system; a part of the peripheral nervous system.

10. Tenth cranial nerve (X) that serves the muscles of the soft palate, pharynx, and larynx, a part of the ear skin, and many organs of the thorax and abdomen.

12. Fourth cranial nerve (IV) that serves an eye muscle.

14. Motor nerve that carries information away from the brain or spinal cord to the periphery of the body.

15. Subdivision of the efferent division of the peripheral nervous system that includes all nerves controlling the muscular system and external sensory receptors.

20. Eleventh cranial nerve (XI) that serves the trapezius and sternocleidomastoid muscles, as well as muscles of the soft palate and pharynx.

24. If it involves the face, there is loss of action of the facial muscles.

25. Division of the brainstem that is involved with the regulation of heartbeat, breathing, vasoconstriction, and reflex centers.

26. Division of the brainstem that includes relay stations for hearing, vision, and motor pathways.

Down

2. Supply of nerves to a tissue or an organ.

3. Division of the central nervous system that runs along the dorsal side of the body and links the brain to the rest of the body.

5. First cranial nerve (I) that transmits smell from the nose to the brain.

6. Junction between two neurons or between a neuron and an effector organ, where neural impulses are transmitted by electrical or chemical means.

7. Cellular component of the nervous system that is individually composed of a cell body and neural processes.

11. Second division of the sensory root of the trigeminal nerve that is formed by the convergence of many nerves, including the infraorbital nerve, and serves varying maxillary tissue, such as the maxillary sinus, palate, nasopharynx, and overlying skin.

13. Sensory nerve that carries information from the periphery of the body to the brain or spinal cord.

16. Sixth cranial nerve (VI) that serves an eye muscle.

17. Largest division of the brain; it coordinates sensory data and motor functions, as well as governing many aspects of intelligence and reasoning, learning and memory.

18 Seventh cranial nerve (VII) that serves the muscles of facial expression.

19. Foramen in the sphenoid bone that carries the trigeminal or fifth cranial nerve.

21. Afferent nerve that carries information from the periphery of the body to the brain or spinal cord.

22. Foramen in the sphenoid bone for the mandibular division of the trigeminal or fifth cranial nerve.

23. Second cranial nerve (II) that transmits sight from the eye to the brain.

CHAPTER 9: ANATOMY OF LOCAL ANESTHESIA

Crossword Puzzle 9

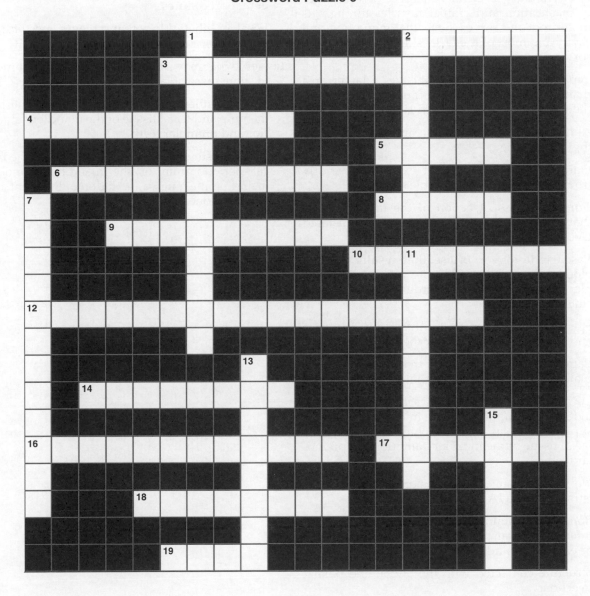

Across

2. Local anesthetic block that achieves anesthesia of the facial tissue of the mandibular premolars and anterior teeth.

3. The loss of feeling or sensation resulting from the use of certain drugs or gases that serve as inhibitory neurotransmitters.

4. Fifth cranial nerve (V) that serves the muscles of mastication and cranial muscles through its motor root and serves the teeth, tongue, and oral cavity and most of the facial skin through its sensory root.

5. Type of injection that anesthetizes a larger area than the local infiltration because the local anesthetic agent is deposited near large nerve trunks.

6. Abnormal sensation from an area, such as burning or prickling.

8. Plate of the mandible that extends superiorly from the body of the mandible.

9. Temporary loss of action of the facial muscles that can occur with an improperly administered IA block.

10. Vascular lesion or bruise that results when a blood vessel is injured and a small amount of blood escapes into the surrounding tissue and clots.

12. Space that is a part of the infratemporal space and that is the target site for the IA block.

14. Paired bones of the skull that consist of two plates, a vertical and a horizontal.

16. Local anesthetic block that achieves anesthesia in the tissue supplied by the middle and anterior superior alveolar nerves, including the pulp and facial tissue of the maxillary anterior and premolar teeth.

17. Nerve anesthetized by diffusion with the administration of the IA block.

18. Bone that contains the foramen that allows the inferior alveolar nerve and blood vessels to exit or enter the mandibular canal.

19. Structure contacted with the buccal and palatal injections.

Down

1. Type of injection that anesthetizes a small area, one or two teeth and associated structures when the local anesthetic agent is deposited near smaller terminal nerve branches off the larger nerve trunks

2. Less dense facial bone than that of the mandible and with less variations, which is injected before dental procedures.

7. Local anesthetic block that achieves anesthesia of the anterior part of the hard palate.

11. Nerve that may serve the mandibular first molar in some cases of failure with the IA block.

13. Local anesthetic block that achieves anesthesia of the pulp and facial tissue of the mandibular anterior and premolar teeth.

15. Local anesthetic block for anesthesia of the buccal periodontium of the mandibular molars, including the gingiva, periodontal ligament, and alveolar bone.

CHAPTER 10: LYMPHATIC SYSTEM

Crossword Puzzle 10

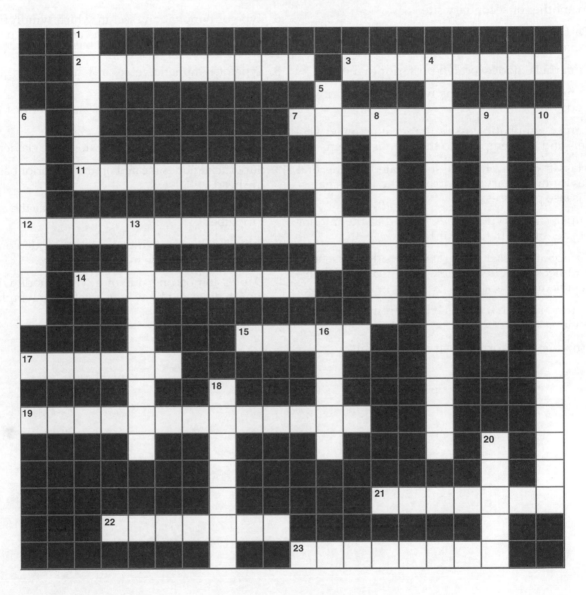

Across

2. Deep cervical nodes located along the accessory nerve.

3. Lymphatic duct draining the lower half of the body and left side of the thorax and also draining the left side of the head and neck through the left jugular trunk.

7. Spread of cancer from the original or primary site to another or secondary site.

11. Part of the immune system with nodes, ducts, tonsils, and vessels.

12. Superficial nodes located posterior to the ear.

14. Lymph node that drains lymph from a primary node.

15. Larger lymphatic vessels that drain smaller vessels and then empty into the venous system.

17. Masses of lymphoid tissue located in the oral cavity and pharynx to protect the body against disease processes.

19. Superficial cervical nodes located at the inferior border of the mandibular ramus.

21. Lymphatic vessel that drains one side of the head and neck and then empties into that side's lymphatic duct.

22. Lymph node that drains lymph from a particular region.

23. Another term for the pharyngeal tonsils.

Down

1. Superficial nodes located along the facial vein that include the malar, nasolabial, buccal, and mandibular nodes.

4. Deep nodes located near the deep parotid nodes and at the level of the first cervical vertebra.

5. System of channels that drains tissue fluid from the surrounding regions.

6. Type of lymphatic vessel in which lymph flows out of the lymph node in the area of the node's hilus.

8. Type of lymphatic vessel in which lymph flows into the lymph node.

9. Superficial cervical nodes located inferior to the chin.

10. Deep cervical nodes located along the clavicle.

13. Superficial nodes located on the posterior base of the head.

16. Tonsil located in the nasopharynx near the auditory tube.

18. Indistinct layer of lymphoid tissue located on the dorsal surface of the tongue's base.

20. Depression on one side of a lymph node where lymph flows out by way of an efferent lymphatic vessel.

CHAPTER 11: FASCIAE AND SPACES

Crossword Puzzle 11

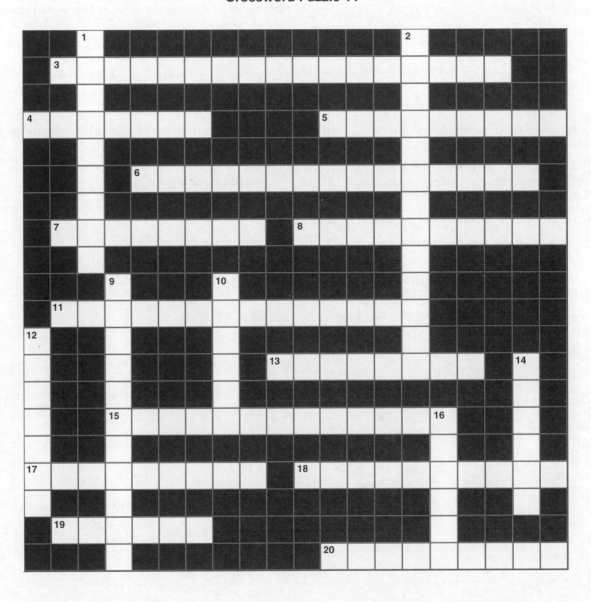

Across

3. Space that is a part of the infratemporal space.

4. Sheath of deep cervical fasciae forming a tube running down the side of the neck.

5. Space located midline between the mandibular symphysis and hyoid bone.

6. Deep cervical fasciae that encloses the entire upper part of the alimentary canal.

7. Deep cervical fasciae that is a single midline tube running down the neck.

8. Space that includes the entire area of the mandible and muscles of mastication.

11. Fascial space located lateral to the pharynx.

13. Deep fascia covering the temporalis muscle down to the zygomatic arch.

15. Space located between the masseter muscle and external surface of the vertical mandibular ramus.

17. Most external layer of the deep cervical fasciae.

18. Space located deep to the oral mucosa, thus making this tissue its roof.

19. Potential spaces between the layers of fasciae in the body.

20. Deep cervical fasciae that cover the vertebrae, spinal column, and associated muscles.

Down

1. Deep fasciae located on the medial surface of the medial pterygoid muscle.

2. Space located lateral and posterior to the submental space on each side of the jaws.

9. Fascial space located between the visceral and investing fasciae.

10. Layers of fibrous connective tissue that underlie the skin and surround the muscles, bones, vessels, nerves, organs, and other structures of the body.

12. Fascial space created inside the investing fascial layer of the deep cervical fasciae as it envelops the parotid salivary gland.

14. Fascial space between buccinator and masseter muscles.

16. Fascial space located lateral to the apex of the maxillary canine.

CHAPTER 12: SPREAD OF INFECTION

Crossword Puzzle 12

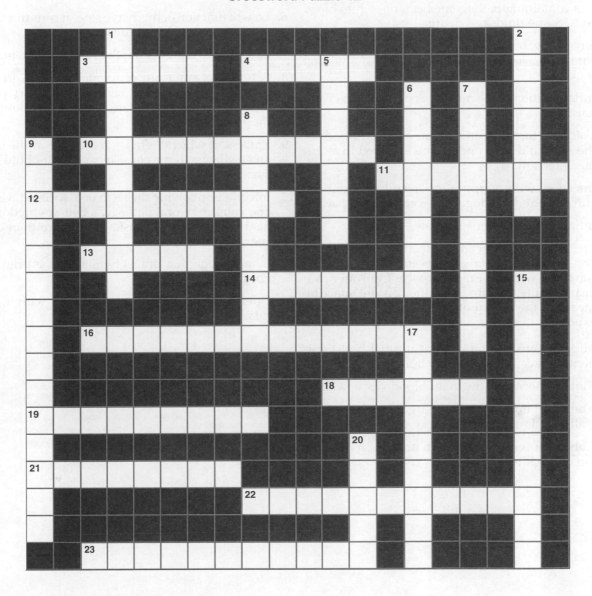

Across

3. Most of these involving the face have one-way valves like the rest of the circulatory system.

4. The route of dental infection traveling through these structures varies according to the teeth involved.

10. Pus containing pathogenic bacteria, white blood cells, tissue fluid, and debris.

11. Small elevated well- circumscribed suppuration-containing lesion of either the skin or the oral mucosa.

12. Inflammation of the meninges of the brain or spinal cord.

13. This structure is located on the side of the body of the sphenoid bone and can be involved in a serious infection.

14. Infection with suppuration resulting from the entrapment of pathogens in a contained space.

16. Inflammation of bone marrow.

18. These allow the spread of infection from the teeth and associated oral tissue because the pathogens can travel within the fascial spaces from one space near the infected site to another distant space by means of the spread of the related inflammatory exudate.

19. Microorganisms that are not normal body residents and can cause an infection.

21. Clot that forms on the inner blood vessel wall.

22. Abnormal hole in a hollow organ, such as in the wall of a sinus.

23. Abnormal sensation from an area, such as burning or prickling.

Down

1. Diffuse inflammation of soft tissue.

2. Passageway in the skin, mucosa, or even bone allowing drainage of an abscess at the surface.

5. Foreign material or thrombus traveling in the blood that can block the vessel.

6. Loss of function of this nerve since it runs through the cavernous sinus, results in paralysis.

7. Bacteria traveling within the vascular system.

8. Secondary sinusitis of dental origin occurs mainly in these sinuses, since the maxillary posterior teeth and associated tissue are close to these sinuses.

9. Process in which there is an increase in the size and a change in the consistency of lymphoid tissue.

15. Infections involving the teeth or associated tissue and caused by oral pathogens that are predominantly anaerobic and usually of more than one species.

17. Lymph node that drains lymph from a primary node.

20. Opening, such as that which occurs with a fistula.

PART 3: CHAPTER WORD SEARCHES

CHAPTER 3. SKELETAL SYSTEM

Words to Find

ANGLE	INFRAORBITAL	PALATINE	SULCUS
ARCH	INFRATEMPORAL	PERFORATION	SUTURE
ARTICULATION	JUGULAR	PROTUBERANCE	SYMPHYSIS
BODY	LACRIMAL	RIM	TEMPORAL
CONCHA	LINE	SAGITTAL	TUBEROSITY
CONDYLE	MAXILLA	SPHENOID	VERTEBRAE
CREST	MEATUS	SPINE	ZYGOMATIC
EMINENCE	NASION	STYLOMASTOID	
FORAMEN	OCCIPITAL	SUBLINGUAL	
HAMULUS	PALATE	SUBMANDIBULAR	

Word Search Puzzle 1

```
U L V E R T E B R A E M Y I R W M F I N
K C S Y M P H Y S I S C H N S I S G A D
F A A K N Z N A S I O N O F U N U A P F
F W J U G U L A R J O P C R B C B S E O
V C O N D Y L E T I K V C A L I M H R R
S T Y L O M A S T O I D I T I S A F T A
S P A L A T E A W S L W P E N U N B U M
P J S G M F R A D C A M I M G R D L R E
H F A K H O C R I L C E T P U A I S E N
E W L V F E L T L U R A A O A E B A T R
N F T R L N A I U U I T L R L G U G U L
O V E G E M X C N C S M U M A W I L I B P
I P N Y O A A U U E A S T L Z R A T E A
D A D G M V J L U N L S P I N E R T R L
S O Y I N F R A O R B I T A L T Y A O A
B Z A Y P R O T U B E R A N C E L L S T
S U L C U S O I H C O N C H A J N X I I
N R C R E S T O K T E M P O R A L L T N
D S U T U R E N D H A M U L U S K F Y E
F R I M M D E M I N E N C E G A R C H A
```

CHAPTER 4: MUSCULAR SYSTEM

Words to Find

ACTION
BUCCINATOR
CERVICAL
CONTRACTION
DEPRESSION
DIGASTRIC
GENIOGLOSSUS
GENIOHYOID

HEAD
HYOGLOSSUS
HYPERTROPHY
INFRAHYOID
INSERTION
MASTICATION
MUSCLE
MUSCULAR

ORIGIN
PALATE
PALATOGLOSSUS
PHARYNX
PLATYSMA
PROTRUSION
RETRACTION
STYLOGLOSSUS

STYLOPHARYNGEUS
SUPRAHYOID
SWALLOWING
TEMPORALIS
TRAPEZIUS
TRIGEMINAL
ZYGOMATICUS

Word Search Puzzle 2

```
A Q C E R V I C A L V P M U S C U L A R
I N F R A H Y O I D S U A M U S C L E L
Z S J V Z Y M N I I P G S L A C T I O N
H T S P A Q P O H G A E T K A V C Q O Z
Z Y T H T M A R E A L N I K P T I D C E
B L Y A R A I I A S A I C N I S E E Q T
U O L R A K P G D T T O A I R Z S P V V
C P O Y P M E I L R O G T C Y Y U R R T
C H G N E C C N H I G L I R C G P E S R
I A L X Z I H G P C L O O E O O R S W I
N R O T I N Y E R H O S N R N M A S A G
A Y S E U S P N O Y S S P E T A H I L E
T N S M S E E I T O S U L T R T Y O L M
O G U P H R R O R G U S A R A I O N O I
R E S O X T T H U L S W T A C C I A W N
P U Y R I I R Y S O Q E Y C T U D Q I A
Z S A A E O O O I S O P S T I S S E N L
I K L L R N P I O S A K M I O F N N G B
Z E P I J P H D N U J B A O N P U R L C
C X I S P C Y T H S P O P N M Y G R D Q
```

CHAPTER 5: TEMPOROMANDIBULAR JOINT

Words to Find

CAPSULE	ELEVATION	POSTGLENOID	SYNOVIAL
CAVITIES	EMINENCE	PROTRUSION	TEMPORAL
CONDYLE	FLUID	PTERYGOID	TEMPORALIS
CONTRACTION	FOSSA	RETRACTION	TRIGEMINAL
DEPRESSION	GLIDING	ROTATION	
DISC	MANDIBLE	STYLOMANDIBULAR	
DISORDER	MOVEMENTS	SUBLUXATION	

Word Search Puzzle 3

```
I W M R W S U B L U X A T I O N Z F L P
O N A R C O N D Y L E C L N K O X M W L
N P N E B T P X F D F L U I D F O S S A
D R D D X S O E M I N E N C E Z D H S U
E O I U W U S T N P G Y S Y N O V I A L
P T B T U S T W K C O N T R A C T I O N
R R L F B B G M O V E M E N T S U X Y R
E U E S T Y L O M A N D I B U L A R F W
S S R E P X E E N V T E M P O R A L L W
S I Q N C T N Z R N R P N A R U V A U G
I O E S A W O T M Y H O D K C I N Y N N
O N K W V A I X W C I R T M S I W I U Y
N E J H I D D A L T O G O A M S D P Z H
W C S I T I P H C E I K T E T I R Q Q H
U A F K I S R A J D A Q G X L I V V O D
H P W X E C R C Y X J I W G H V O S J M
O S D V S T E M P O R A L I S I T N T X
S U X Z E Y A T P T P T E R Y G O I D S
B L A R D I S O R D E R N A M X Z L C S
K E T E L E V A T I O N L K T O M O Y I
```

CHAPTER 6: VASCULAR SYSTEM

Words to Find

ANASTOMOSIS	HEMATOMA	PLEXUS	VEIN
ARTERIOLE	HEMORRHAGE	PTERYGOID	VENOUS
ARTERY	INCISIVE	PULSE	VENULE
BACTEREMIA	INFRAORBITAL	RETROMANDIBULAR	
BRACHIOCEPHALIC	LINGUAL	SINUSES	
CAROTID	MAXILLARY	SUBCLAVIAN	
EMBOLUS	MENTAL	SUBLINGUAL	
FACIAL	OCCIPITAL	THROMBUS	

Word Search Puzzle 4

```
V E N O U S F A C I A L O M E N T A L Z
K Q V P A N A S T O M O S I S P R N X W
M N N R M E K B A C T E R E M I A C C E
V A R T E R I O L E P I K Y X N L I B B
Z R C Z Y T H O C C I P I T A L L Q Y Q
S Z F Q M I R Z A R T E R Y F A K C U T
A U A E A K N O D Y X F T R H N K S A S
T V B V X N F F M S B E W P C G Y I H U
H E M C I P Y W R A G I E B P T Y N E B
R I P U L S E F V A N C S E G H S U M L
O N V L L A C V H Y O D P A Q U R S A I
M L G K A R V R Z I N R I L Z H E E T N
B I L B R K R I H N Q J B B E L E S O G
U N N W Y O T C A D Q F S I U X S Q M U
S G N K M N A K I N L U M N T L U C A A
E U Z E U R E T G T L I E F S A A S O L
T A H M B T O G P O M V G V V K L R C J
P L R S R R R S M B Z P T E R Y G O I D
B Z S X A C B M U T M X M M N T G D L N
N A X C D M E O I N C I S I V E A K K L
```

CHAPTER 7: GLANDULAR TISSUE

Words to Find

CARUNCLE
DUCT
ENDOCRINE
EXOCRINE
GLAND
GOITER

LACRIMAL
MAJOR
MINOR
MUCOCELE
MUMPS
PARATHYROID

PAROTID
RANULA
SALIVA
STONE
SUBLINGUAL
SUBMANDIBULAR

THYMUS
THYROID
THYROXINE

Word Search Puzzle 5

```
Z G O I T E R N B D D Z Z S E M T R H Q
M Q F S N C G L A N D D P A Y N T M D T
I A B C A R U N C L E B G L X E N V Q E
R S U B L I N G U A L W D I M V F T U V
A I W Z X G B Q R G D E X V W X S R X V
N Q N Z R O X L A C R I M A L F O W B J
U T H Y R O X I N E X D C R Y J I V S W
L I E S U B M A N D I B U L A R A J R X
A G N P V K N Q X T E O T M I H U M A W
D I D A X A A L O J O C T H Y M U S N H
H E O R V H J R V N U M U C O C E L E B
H Y C A Q B A T I D Z Q M I N O R S N E
A I R T Z P B I P B R U N A C F C X S E
E E I H H N N A O S L A C R I M A L Y N
V Q N Y S T O N E X O C R I N E M O L L
Q U E R S U M N S G W P D G P M U D G B
L B Z O O X I J S S K X Y B Y I M E L D
R T S I J Y W C J V Y S M W V J P H W F
S O T D Y D O L Y M P H C Y T E S U M Z
T H Y R O I D P E N S L V G V V W R R J
```

CHAPTER 8: NERVOUS SYSTEM

Words to Find

ABDUCENS	DIENCEPHALON	MEDULLA	PONS
AFFERENT	FACIAL	NERVE	ROTUNDUM
ANESTHESIA	GANGLION	NEURON	SENSORY
AUTONOMIC	HYPOGLOSSAL	OCULOMOTOR	THALAMUS
BRAIN	HYPOTHALAMUS	OPTIC	TROCHLEAR
BRAINSTEM	INNERVATION	OVALE	VAGUS
CEREBELLUM	MANDIBULAR	PARALYSIS	
CORD	MAXILLARY	PERIPHERAL	

Word Search Puzzle 6

```
C J A H T H A L A M U S S C P T L A X P
F D W A S E N S O R Y U E W V I F T D R
H N E R V E R W A T M O P T I C M C M X
Q P E R I P H E R A L V O V A L E Y A J
C M E K U J L O L P A R A L Y S I S N J
P K Q O W H N A B D U C E N S E P A D T
O N J U C S H E M V A G U S N O M N I Y
L C E O O T Q H Y P O G L O S S A L B M
A S R U O M E D U L L A I I Z V X E U O
F T S P R W L I Y K V T Z A I F I L L C
A I Y W B O Z E V Y A E V N V D L T A U
C H B K P A N N Z V C D O Y D E L I R L
T A R A O U Z C R O R I E L B E A S U O
O J A F N T Q E E O L L S E M T R R G M
R P I F S O N P C G H U R O L D Y U I O
Y D N E L N V H N A N E S T H E S I A T
F H T R I O S A W O C F A C I A L J W O
C K J E K M G L B R A I N S T E M I X R
H K H N V I H O Y E G W T R Y X J P W I
H H J T V C K N U J H R O T U N D U M O
```

CHAPTER 9: ANATOMY OF LOCAL ANESTHETIC

Words to Find

ANESTHESIA
BLOCK
BONE
BUCCAL
HEMATOMA

INCISIVE
INFILTRATION
INFRAORBITAL
LINGUAL
MANDIBLE

MAXILLA
MENTAL
MYLOHYOID
NASOPALATINE
PALATINE

PARALYSIS
PARESTHESIA
RAMUS
TRIGEMINAL

Word Search Puzzle 7

```
J U T S D O P K C W A N E S T H E S I A
B C R H U M C I N C I S I V E O V L P K
A P I S X R Q N G W W A G L Z U H I W Y
Y K G O F P O F P A L A T I N E Z N T E
N X E V R D N I B L V B U N D A J G Y G
P Q M Q R Y Y L N M C I W T J N R U R L
A K I C S Z L T I H E O Y A T A Y A J N
R I N F R A O R B I T A L J T S H L R B
E P A T C C T A X N F Z N F X O D A U B
S K L C M E N T A L G W T K A P J D R D L
T L U F H B S I H E M A T O M A H S I O
H B S O B I O O C F S T J M A L M Y U C
E R R P D R V N T S T J F A F A O N S K
S A K T F P A Q E C B I Z X D T S O L F
I Z H U K K P A R A L Y S I S I F H F Y
A M Y F N N K T U C V B H L J N P W O C W
S K L M Y L O H Y O I D F L G E L N I R
C A R A M U S A E V U P M A R G P P C J
E K P N M F D I T I A L U F V Q Y O T E
W N A M A N D I B L E W B Q D A P N T O
```

CHAPTER 10: LYMPHATIC SYSTEM

Words to Find

ACCESSORY
ADENOIDS
AFFERENT
DUCTS
EFFERENT
FACIAL
HILUS

JUGULAR
JUGULODIGASTRIC
LINGUAL
LYMPH
LYMPHADENOPATHY
LYMPHATICS
METASTASIS

NODES
OCCIPITAL
PALATINE
PRIMARY
RETROAURICULAR
RETROPHARYNGEAL
SECONDARY

SUBMANDIBULAR
SUBMENTAL
SUPRACLAVICULAR
THORACIC
TONSIL
TUBAL
VESSELS

Word Search Puzzle 8

```
H F Z S T H I L U S E C O N D A R Y C I
S A K J U G U L A R X I Z S W I S H I P
J F A S J L Y M P H A T I C S T X G T T
Z F C T O W G X N T E D O O G F O B O F
V E O C C I P I T A L O E P C L Z A N J
I R B F A C I A L B X B Q N F N S C S U
Y E U Q D Z D U C T S C E C O O L C I G
G N C N O D E S V Y A K Y M O I Q E L U
G T E Y R T K T P A L A T I N E D S I L
Q S U B M A N D I B U L A R T Q O S L O
O Y R E T R O A U R I C U L A R P O J D
A A B S U P R A C L A V I C U L A R C I
E Q Q R S U B M E N T A L B O L D Y D G
B P R I M A R Y X E V B M K A K D A S A
X F L D R E T R O P H A R Y N G E A L S
Y R Y X U V E S S E L S T U B A L L M T
O N C L Y M P H A D E N O P A T H Y I R
A T E F F E R E N T L I N G U A L M Z I
N T Z I J M E T A S T A S I S X N P H C
J V G B W C U F H T H O R A C I C H F N
```

CHAPTER 11: FASCIAE AND SPACES

Words to Find

BUCCAL	INVESTING	RETROPHARYNGEAL	TEMPORAL
BUCCOPHARYNGEAL	MASTICATOR	SPACES	VERTEBRAL
CANINE	PARAPHARYNGEAL	SUBLINGUAL	VISCERAL
CAROTID	PAROTID	SUBMANDIBULAR	
FASCIA	PREVISCERAL	SUBMASSETERIC	
INFRATEMPORAL	PTERYGOID	SUBMENTAL	

Word Search Puzzle 9

```
Y J I I X R F Y P W X P M M P A W S I V
Z B N B O V A Z A M E R A L A C O U N I
F U V N Y Q S W R M P E S W R V L B F S
A C E J G D C C A I R T T E O L B M R C
R C S Z V D I J P I E R I B T C W E A E
A O T I Q I A F H C V O C U I A V N T R
U P I O P U X N A A I P A C D R E T E A
O H N H G Z F E R N S H T C S O R A M L
H A G C Y S N W Y I C A O A B T T L P W
J R M D D P V J N N E R R L K I E V O J
V Y N R B A E U G E R Y T J B D B Z R S
H N B S L C Z A E G A N E X F S R X A O
T G L S I E V W A H L G R D C J A P L N
U E R C S S E M L W H E B U J I L P O Z
U A R Z H Z D S U B M A S S E T E R I C
L L N G X M Q Q S U B L I N G U A L W G
L S U B M A N D I B U L A R L P O U P Y
F U J H U W F S V A U R N O H K O H J V
Y I T M R Z F P T E R Y G O I D R D M P
J W V G T E M P O R A L C Y G T G X G Q
```

CHAPTER 12: SPREAD OF INFECTION

Words to Find

ABDUCENS	MAXILLARY	PATHOGENS	STOMA
ABSCESS	MENINGITIS	PERFORATION	SUPPURATION
BACTEREMIA	NODES	PRIMARY	THROMBUS
CELLULITIS	ODONTOGENIC	PUSTULE	VEINS
EMBOLUS	OPPORTUNISTIC	SECONDARY	
FISTULA	OSTEOMYELITIS	SINUS	
LYMPHADENOPATHY	PARESTHESIA	SPACES	

Word Search Puzzle 10

```
B M R Q I M E C K U J C U L D P S T L G
A S U A B D U C E N S E X I P U C H Y F
C B P N W M T A E L F V H L Y S Y R M I
T B D A J G O O Z V L C T R N T K O P T
E N A I C M N S N N A U A Z A U V M H E
R C B O S E R S T Q D M L J M L T B A J
E Q S G G N S V C E I S S I N E C U D F
M U C S E I T T P R O I I O T A P S E I
I S E E X N H I P B M M I N I I X V N S
A U S C Z G B T C X O T Y S U U S T O T
X P S O E I G L I M A P E E N S Q L P U
H P J N P T J S P R Z H N L L P K S A L
X U S D E I O D O N T O G E N I C J T A
S R C A S S P F R S W P C S X F T E H P
B A O R H T R B E W J J X E P B Q I Y C
V T N Y R E O R A O Z W E M B O L U S N
E I A O P H A M M A X I L L A R Y O J O
I O J A T P A Z A F Z W T N Z R T I C D
N N P O P P O R T U N I S T I C O C X E
S X T C Z Z Z L P A T H O G E N S M E S
```

CHAPTER 1: INTRODUCTION TO HEAD AND NECK ANATOMY

Note: Answers can be obtained from your instructor and their Evolve Resources unless from textbook source.

Matching

Match each item below with its best short description; each single item can only be matched once.

a.	Dorsal	k.	Superficial	u.	Median section
b.	Axial plane	l.	Internal	v.	Frontal section
c.	Midsagittal plane	m.	Apex	w.	Variation
d.	External	n.	Coronal plane	x.	Distal
e.	Deep	o.	Transverse plane	y.	Inferior
f.	Posterior	p.	Median	z.	Ipsilateral
g.	Contralateral	q.	Lateral		
h.	Ventral	r.	Anatomic position		
i.	Anterior	s.	Superior		
j.	Anatomic nomenclature	t.	Medial		

1. System of names for anatomic structures _____

2. The body can be standing erect _____

3. Front of an area _____

4. Back of an area _____

5. Part directed toward anterior _____

6. Part directed toward posterior _____

7. Area faces toward head _____

8. Area faces toward feet _____

9. Pointed end of conical structure _____

10. Divided into equal right and left halves _____

11. Divided into anterior and posterior parts _____

12. Divided into superior and inferior parts _____

13. Located at median plane _____

14. Area closer to midsagittal plane _____

15. Area farther away from median plane _____

16. Dental term for area away from median plane _____

17. On same side of body _____

18. Opposite side of body _____

19. Toward the surface _____

20. Inward away from surface _____

21. Inner side of wall _____

22. Outer side of wall _____

23. Division by midsagittal plane _____

24. Division by coronal plane _____

25. Division by transverse plane _____

26. Specific anatomic details are not the same _____

True or False

Assign the statement below as either true or false. For deeper understanding, edit the false statements until they are true.

1. An understanding of anatomy helps determine pathologic lesions. _____

2. It is important to know the infection source as well as where it could spread. _____

3. The administration of local anesthesia is only based on the teeth. _____

4. Anatomic position is the system of names for anatomic structures. _____

5. Anatomic nomenclature has the patient always supine in the dental chair. _____

6. A part directed toward the posterior is considered ventral. _____

7. The back of an area is considered its posterior part. _____

8. The area that faces toward the feet is considered internal. _____

9. The apex can also be considered the tip of the conical structure. _____

10. A midsagittal plane is also considered to be a median plane. _____

11. A sagittal plane is always perpendicular to the median plane. _____

12. The coronal plane is also considered to be a midsagittal plane. _____

13. The structure at the median plane is considered to be median. _____

14. Dental term for a structure being closer to the midsagittal plane is distal. _____

15. Dental term for a structure being away from the midsagittal plane is mesial. _____

16. The ears are lateral to the eyes on the face. _____

17. The fingers are distal of the same side shoulder. _____

18. The right leg is contralateral to the right arm. _____

19. The skin is deep to the bones and the bones are superficial to the skin. _____

20. A transverse section is also considered to be an axial section. _____

21. A sagittal section can also be considered a mid-sagittal section. _____

22. A coronal section can also be considered a frontal section. _____

23. A median section can also be considered a frontal section. _____

24. Joints and nerves can vary in a patient. _____

25. The number of bones in a patient is usually constant. _____

CHAPTER 2: SURFACE ANATOMY

Note: Answers can be obtained from your instructor and their Evolve Resources unless from textbook source.

Matching

Match each item below with its best short description; each single item can only be matched once.

a.	Nasal septum	k.	Sulcus terminalis	u.	Labiomental groove
b.	Zygomatic arch	l.	Foramen cecum	v.	Lingual tonsil
c.	Vertical dimensions of the face	m.	Nasolabial sulcus	w.	Plica fimbriata
d.	Labial commissure	n.	Sublingual caruncle	x.	Retromolar pad
e.	Glabella	o.	External acoustic meatus	y.	Maxillary tuberosity
f.	Frontal region	p.	Root of the nose	z.	Frontal eminence
g.	Sublingual fold	q.	Lingual frenum		
h.	Supraorbital ridge	r.	Pterygomandibular fold		
i.	Bridge of the nose	s.	Surface anatomy		
j.	Palatine rugae	t.	Temple		

1. Structural relationships of external features to internal organs and parts _____

2. Region that includes forehead and area superior to the eyes _____

3. Structure directly inferior to each eyebrow _____

4. Smooth elevated area between the eyebrows _____

5. Prominence of the forehead _____

6. Superficial side of the head posterior to each eye _____

7. Tube through which sound waves are transmitted _____

8. Part of nasal region located between the eyes _____

9. Bony structure inferior to nasion _____

10. Separates nares within the midline _____

11. Structure of the cheekbone _____

12. Dividing the face into thirds _____

13. Corner of the mouth at each end _____

14. Groove running upward between labial commissure and ala _____

15. Structure on mandible just posterior to most distal mandibular molar _____

16. Elevation on maxilla just posterior to most distal maxillary molar _____

17. Firm irregular ridges of tissue directly posterior to incisive papilla _____

18. Vertical fold of tissue that runs from incisive papilla to uvula _____

19. Anterior midline fold between ventral tongue and floor of mouth _____

20. Ridge of tissue on each side of the floor of mouth _____

21 Small papilla at anterior end of each sublingual fold _____

22. Fringe-like projections lateral to each deep lingual veins on each side _____

23. A V-shaped groove separating base from body of the tongue _____

24. Small pitlike depression on dorsal surface of the tongue _____

25. Irregular mass of lymphoid tissue on dorsal surface of tongue _____

26. Groove that separates lower lip from the chin _____

True or False

Assign the statement below as either true or false. For deeper understanding, edit the false statements until they are true.

1. Labiomental groove is almost midway between apex of the nose and chin. _____

2. The angle of the mandible is inferior to the ear's lobule. _____

3. Structures closer to the inner cheek are considered palatal. _____

4. The buccal mucosa covers the inner parts of the lips. _____

5. Those structures closest to the tongue are termed facial. _____

6. The parotid papilla is just opposite the mandibular second molar. _____

7. Mucogingival junction is between the attached gingiva and alveolar mucosa. _____

8. The nonattached gingiva at the gingival margin is the marginal gingiva. _____

9. The inner surface of the marginal gingiva faces the gingival sulcus. _____

10. The interdental papilla is an extension of interdental gingiva between teeth. _____

11. Mandibular anterior teeth overlap the maxillary anterior teeth. _____

12. The alveolar mucosa is redder and thinner than the labial mucosa. _____

13. The alveolar process is the bony extension for the mandible. _____

14. The labial frena are folds of tissue between the labial and alveolar mucosa. _____

15. The vestibules between the lips and cheeks are diamond-shaped. _____

16. The midline of the upper lip ends in tubercle. _____

17. The philtrum is a horizontal groove superior to the midline of the upper lip. _____

18. The masseter muscle is felt when a person relaxes their teeth apart. _____

19. The nares are another term for nostrils. _____

20. The alae of the nose are found laterally on each side. _____

21. The outer corners of the eyes are considered the commissures. _____

22. The conjunctiva line the inside of the eyelids. _____

23. The sclera changes size responding to various light conditions. _____

24. The pupil appears black within the eyeball. _____

25. The tragus is the smaller flap of tissue of the auricle. _____

CHAPTER 3: SKELETAL SYSTEM

Note: Answers can be obtained from your instructor and their Evolve Resources unless from textbook source.

Matching

Match each item below with its best short description; each single item can only be matched once.

a.	Tuberosity	k.	Bone	u.	Fracture
b.	Arch	l.	Ostium	v.	Meatus
c.	Fovea	m.	Articulation	w.	Joint
d.	Plate	n.	Tubercle	x.	Fossa
e.	Crest	o.	Sulcus	y.	Cornu
f.	Spine	p.	Condyle	z.	Suture
g.	Canal	q.	Head		
h.	Process	r.	Aperture		
i.	Line	s.	Foramen		
j.	Notch	t.	Fissure		

1. Any prominence on bony surface _____

2. Specific type of prominence on bony surface _____

3. Rounded projection from bony surface _____

4. Large rough prominence on bony surface _____

5. Prominence shaped like a bridge _____

6. Hornlike prominence on bony surface _____

7. Small rounded eminence on bony surface _____

8. Prominent border or ridge on bony surface _____

9. Straight ridge on bony surface _____

10. Blunt or sharply pointed projection _____

11. One type of depression with indentation on the edge _____

12. Groove for blood vessels or nerves on bony surface _____

13. Generally deeper depression on bony surface _____

14. Pitlike depression on bony surface that is small _____

15. Flat structure of a bone _____

16. Opening like a window in bone _____

17. Narrow and cleftlike opening in bone _____

18. Smaller opening in bone into a hollow organ or canal _____

19. Narrow opening in bone _____

20. Type of canal in bone _____

21. Longer narrow tubelike opening in bone _____

22. Area where bones are joined to each other _____

23. Union between two or more bones _____

24. Union of bones with a jagged line _____

25. Broken bone due to physical force _____

26. Mineralized structure protecting the internal soft tissue _____

True or False

Assign the statement below as either true or false. For deeper understanding, edit the false statements until they are true.

1. The bony prominences and depressions serve as nerve attachments. _____

2. The facial bones create the cranium. _____

3. Growth in lower face takes place at bony surfaces of the mandible. _____

4. At the anterior part of the skull is the single frontal bone. _____

5. At the posterior part of the skull is the single occipital bone. _____

6. Anterior fontanelle joins the frontal bone and only one parietal bone. _____

7. Paired sagittal suture extends from anterior skull to posterior at midline. _____

8. The lambdoidal suture is more serrated-looking than the others. _____

9. The orbit has four walls and an apex. _____

10. The ethmoid bone forms the greatest part of the medial wall of the orbit. _____

11. The orbital apex is composed of the sphenoid bone and palatine bone. _____

12. Medial to the optic canals is the superior orbital fissure. _____

13. The inferior orbital fissure is between the sphenoid bone and the maxilla. _____

14. The frontal and zygomatic bones as well as maxilla form the orbital rim. _____

15. The prominent anterior opening of the nasal cavity is the piriform aperture. _____

16. The choanae are large deeper posterior openings of the nasal cavities. _____

17. Each lateral wall of the nasal cavity has three turbinates. _____

18. The posterior part of the nasal septum is formed by the vomer. _____

19. A deviated nasal septum may be present at birth. _____

20. During the lateral ceph, the Frankfort plane is aligned horizontally. _____

21. The patient that receives a CBCT also needs a panoramic radiograph. _____

22. Transverse palatine suture is between maxillae and palatine bones. _____

23. Each pterygoid process consists of medial and lateral plates. _____

24. The hamulus is superior to the medial plate of pterygoid process. _____

25. The larger anterior opening on the sphenoid bone is the foramen ovale. _____

26. The foramen spinosum carries the middle meningeal artery. _____

27. The carotid canal is an opening in the petrous part of the temporal bone. _____

28. The facial nerve exits the skull by way of the stylomastoid foramen. _____

29. The largest opening on the superior of the skull is the foramen magnum. _____

30. The jugular foramen allow passage of the vagus nerve. _____

31. The foramen rotundum allows the passage of the maxillary nerve. _____

32. The hypoglossal canal allows the passage for the vestibulocochlear nerve. _____

33. The occipital bone can be divided into two parts. _____

34. On the lateral part of the occipital bone are two condyles. _____

35. The lacrimal fossa is just internal to the lateral part of the supraorbital rim. _____

36. Each temporal bone is composed of three parts. _____

37. Posterior to the external acoustic meatus is the mastoid process. _____

38. Lateral to the mastoid process is the mastoid notch. _____

39. The body of the sphenoid bone contains the sphenoidal sinuses. _____

40. The horizontal plates of the palatine bones form the posterior hard palate. _____

41. Patient may feel soreness when pressing on the infraorbital foramen. _____

42. Mandibular symphysis at the midline on the anterior mandibular surface. _____

43. The mandibular ramus serves as the primary attachment site for muscles. _____

44. Coronoid notch is the most superficial depression on mandibular ramus. _____

45. The retromolar triangle is a bony landmark on the posterior edge. _____

46. The mandibular foramen is the opening of the mandibular canal. _____

47. The lingula overhangs the mandibular foramen on each side. _____

48. With age and tooth loss, the alveolar process mandible becomes resorbed. _____

49. A bifid inferior alveolar nerve may be present in rare cases. _____

50. The mylohyoid groove passes from the mental foramen. _____

Table Completion

Fill in the rest of the table from the indicated textbook table.

Table 3.1 Cranial Bones and Facial Bones

Cranial Bones	Number	Facial bones	Number

Table 3.2 Skull Sutures and Articulations

Sutures	Number	Bony articulations
Coronal sutures		
Frontonasal suture		
Intermaxillary suture		
Lambdoidal suture		
Median palatine suture		
Sagittal suture		

Continued

Table 3.2 Skull Sutures and Articulations—cont'd

Sutures	Number	Bony articulations
Squamosal suture		
Temporozygomatic suture		
Transverse palatine suture		
Zygomaticomaxillary suture		

Table 3.3 Skull Bony Openings and Contents (Partial List)

Bony Opening(s)	Location	Contents for Openings
Foramina ovales		
Foramina rotunda		
Greater palatine foramina		
Incisive foramen		
Infraorbital foramina and canals		
Lesser palatine foramina		
Mandibular foramina		
Mental foramina		

Table 3.4 Skull Processes (Partial List)

Process(es) of Skull	Skull Bone	Associated Structures
Alveolar process		
Alveolar process	Mandible	
Condyloid processes		
Coronoid processes		
Frontal processes	Maxillae	
Palatine processes		
Zygomatic processes	Maxillae	

Table 3.5 Orbital Bones

Part of Each Orbit	Skull Bones
Roof or superior wall	
Medial wall	
Lateral wall	
Floor	
Apex or base	

CHAPTER 4: MUSCULAR SYSTEM

Note: Answers can be obtained from your instructor and their Evolve Resources unless from textbook source.

Matching

Match each item below with its best short description; each single item can only be matched once.

a.	Acute trauma	k.	Left	u.	Mouth prop
b.	Chin	l.	Wasting	v.	Suctioning
c.	Facial nerve	m.	Muscles of mastication	w.	Caregiver
d.	Dysphagia	n.	Atrophy	x.	Facial paralysis
e.	Facial appearance	o.	Superficial fascia	y.	Brain
f.	Tongue	p.	Facial expression	z.	Septum
g.	Action	q.	Hypertrophy		
h.	Mouth droop	r.	Mandible		
i.	Homecare	s.	Insertion		
j.	Origin	t.	Muscle		

1. Shortens under neural control, causing structures of body to move _____

2. End of muscle attached to least moveable structure _____

3. End of muscle attached to more movable structure _____

4. Movement accomplished when muscle fibers contract _____

5. Cervical muscle malfunctions from this cause _____

6. If cervical muscles are malfunctioning, cannot possibly raise this _____

7. Muscles of facial expression are found in this facial tissue _____

8. Damage to seventh cranial nerve results in this sign _____

9. Structure anesthetized with incorrect IA or V-A bloc _____

10. Inability to form this can occur with a stroke _____

11. Muscles of face deeper than muscles of facial expression _____

12. All muscles of mastication attached to this structure _____

13. Masseter muscle with those who clench or grind teeth _____

14. Most seek medical attention with enlarged masseter due to this reason _____

15. Thick vascular mass of voluntary muscle anchored to floor of the mouth _____

16. Divides tongue at midlines into two symmetric halves _____

17. Left side strokes of this structure affect movement on right body side _____

18. Difficulty with swallowing that can impact dental care _____

19. Patient may need this to answer questions with speech impairment _____

20. Side of brain with strokes that affects speech function _____

21. Inability to close the mouth due to associated muscles _____

22. May not be adequate for oral health after facial paralysis _____

23. Tongue in severe cases of mouth droop _____

24. Atrophy of tongue occurs due to this process _____

25. Needed if tongue is more active during dental care _____

26. Lifesaver with mouth droop during dental treatment _____

True or False

Assign the statement below as either true or false. For deeper understanding, edit the false statements until they are true.

1. The SCM muscle divides the neck into anterior and lateral cervical triangles. _____

2. Trapezius muscle is superficial to both anterior and posterior neck surfaces. _____

3. Noting facial expression is part of an extraoral examination. _____

4. Bellies of the epicranial muscle are separated by the aponeurosis. _____

5. The orbicularis oculi muscle encircles the mouth. _____

6. Inability to close the eye can result in dryness and damage. _____

7. Glabellar lines can be alleviated with injections in some cases. _____

8. The facial modiolus is a point of contact where many muscles meet. _____

9. Pterygomandibular raphe is a tendinous band located in the oral cavity. _____

10. Zygomaticus major muscle is medial to the zygomaticus minor muscle. _____

11. The mentalis muscle is superior and medial to the mental nerve. _____

12. The muscles of mastication can work in combination. _____

13. The jaw movements involve mandible and not the rest of the skull. _____

14. The most obvious muscle of mastication is the temporalis muscle. _____

15. The medial pterygoid muscle has two heads due to differing depth. _____

16. The two heads of the lateral pterygoid muscle fused together anteriorly. _____

17. Two groups of the hyoid muscles are based on relationship to hyoid bone. _____

18. Suprahyoid muscles are divided into anterior and posterior groups. _____

19. The digastric muscle has three bellies to demarcate the neck. _____

20. The fibers of the mylohyoid muscle run transversely between the two rami. _____

21. The stylohyoid muscle has one slip that is superficial. _____

22. Geniohyoid muscle is superior to the medial border of mylohyoid muscle. _____

23. The infrahyoid muscles are four pairs of hyoid muscles. _____

24. The omohyoid muscle has two separate bellies. _____

25. The sternohyoid muscle is deep to the thyroid gland. _____

26. Muscles of the tongue can be grouped into intrinsic and extrinsic groups. _____

27. The intrinsic muscles of the tongue all end in *glossus*. _____

28. The muscles of the pharynx are involved in speaking and swallowing. _____

29. There are five paired muscles of the soft palate. _____

30. The muscle of the uvula lies outside of the uvula of the palate. _____

Table Completion

Fill in the rest of the table from the indicated textbook table.

Table 4.1 Muscles of Facial Expression

Muscle	Origin	Insertion
Epicranial		
Orbicularis oculi		
Orbicularis oris		
Buccinator		
Risorius		
Levator labii superioris		
Levator labii superioris alaeque nasi		
Zygomaticus major		
Zygomaticus minor		
Levator anguli oris		
Depressor anguli oris		
Depressor labii inferioris		
Mentalis		
Platysma		
Levator anguli oris		

Table 4.2 Muscles of Facial Expression and Associated Facial Expressions

Muscle	Facial Expression(s)
Epicranial	
Orbicularis oculi	
Corrugator supercilia	
Orbicularis oris	
Buccinator	
Risorius	
Levator labii superioris	
Levator labii superioris alaeque nasi	
Zygomaticus major	
Zygomaticus minor	
Levator anguli oris	
Depressor anguli oris	
Depressor labii inferioris	
Mentalis	
Platysma	

Table 4.3 Muscles of Mastication

Muscle	Origin	Insertion
Masseter		
Temporalis		
Medial pterygoid		
Lateral pterygoid		

Table 4.4 Muscles of Mastication and Associated Mandibular Movements

Muscle	Mandibular Movement(s)
Masseter	Bilateral contraction:
Temporalis	Bilateral contraction of entire muscle: Bilateral contraction of only posterior part:
Medial pterygoid	Bilateral contraction:
Lateral pterygoid	Unilateral contraction: Bilateral contraction:

CHAPTER 5: TEMPOROMANDIBULAR JOINT

Note: Answers can be obtained from your instructor and their Evolve Resources unless from textbook source.

Matching

Match each item below with its best short description; each single item can only be matched once.

a.	Mandibular	k.	Reinforcement	u.	Retraction
b.	Condyle	l.	Meckel	v.	Minor
c.	External carotid	m.	Joint disc	w.	Stylomandibular
d.	Protrusion	n.	Synovial cavities	x.	Capsule
e.	Submandibular	o.	Barrier	y.	Sphenomandibular
f.	Synovial fluid	p.	Mastication	z.	Joint
g.	Cranial	q.	Lingula		
h.	Ligament	r.	Inferior alveolar		
i.	Temporomandibular	s.	Facial		
j.	Superior deep cervical	t.	Pterygoid		

1. Site of junction or union between two or more bones _____

2. Nerve that serves the TMJ by its branches _____

3. Blood supply to TMJ by its one branch _____

4. Motor function for TMJ by these muscles _____

5. Venous return for TMJ includes this plexus _____

6. Lymph from the TMJ is drained deeply into these nodes _____

7. Type of skull bone for superior part of the joint _____

8. Type of skull bone for inferior part of the joint _____

9. Part of mandible surface that articulates in the TMJ _____

10. Fibrous structure that completely encloses the TMJ _____

11. Structure located between the two bones of the TMJ _____

12. Two compartments of the TMJ _____

13. Lubrication of the joint by the capsule _____

14. Band of fibrous tissues that connects bones _____

15. Major ligament of the TMJ _____

16. Variable ligament of the TMJ from area cervical fascia _____

17. Ligament of the TMJ located medial side of mandible _____

18. Sphenomandibular ligament is an embryonic vestige of this cartilage _____

19. Nerve descending between sphenomandibular and mandibular ramus _____

20. Attachment over mandibular foramen by sphenomandibular ligament _____

21. Mandibular movement to accentuate sphenomandibular ligament _____

22. Action of sphenomandibular ligament to agent with incorrect IA block _____

23. Stylomandibular ligament separates parotid gland from other gland _____

24. The TMJ ligament acts as this to the lateral part of the joint capsule _____

25. The TMJ ligament prevents this movement from becoming excessive _____

26. Two of the ligaments of the TMJ that are not major _____

True or False

Assign the statement below as either true or false. For deeper understanding, edit the false statements until they are true.

1. The TMJ allows movement of the mandible for respiratory movements. _____

2. Both articulating bony TMJ surfaces are covered by fibrocartilage. _____

3. The articulating area of the temporal bone is its petrous part. _____

4. The articulating area of the temporal bone includes the articular eminence. _____

5. The articular fossa is anterior to the articular eminence. _____

6. The articular fossa is an oval-shaped depression. _____

7. Posterior to the articular fossa is the postglenoid process. _____

8. The joint disc margins are continuous with the joint capsule. _____

9. On sagittal section, the joint disc appears cap-like. _____

10. Shape of joint disc at no time conforms to the shape of adjoining bones. _____

11. Another name for the joint disc is *Meckel cartilage*. _____

12. An upper and lower synovial cavity divides the TMJ. _____

13. The inner lining of oral mucosa secretes the synovial fluid. _____

14. The synovial fluid is watery, rather like lymph. _____

15. The TMJ gliding movement occurs mainly between disc and articular fossa. _____

16. Bringing the jaw forward involves protrusion of the mandible. _____

17. The TMJ rotational movement occurs mainly between disc and condyle. _____

18. Opening the jaws involves both depression and protrusion of the mandible. _____

19. Closing the jaws involves both elevation and depression of the mandible. _____

20. Lateral deviation of mandible involves shifting the lower jaw to one side. _____

21. Lateral deviation involves both gliding and rotational movements. _____

22. Interocclusal clearance is approximately 10 to 20 mm between the arches. _____

23. Assess the mandible at the TMJ, by placing a finger on the tragus. _____

24. A TMD is a group of musculoskeletal and neuromuscular conditions. _____

25. Most of the symptoms of TMJ originate from muscles supporting the joint. _____

Table Completion

Fill in the rest of the table from the indicated textbook table.

Table 5.1 Mandibular Movements of Temporomandibular Joint and Muscles

Mandibular Movement(s)	Temporomandibular Joint Movement(s)	Associated Muscle(s)
Protrusion of mandible moving mandible forward		
Retraction of mandible moving mandible backward		
Elevation and retraction of mandible closing jaws		
Depression and protrusion of mandible opening jaws		
Lateral deviation of mandible to shift mandible to one side		

CHAPTER 6: VASCULAR SYSTEM

Note: Answers can be obtained from your instructor and their Evolve Resources unless from textbook source.

Matching

Match each item below with its best short description; each single item can only be matched once.

a.	Artery	k.	Network	u.	Aorta
b.	Arterial	l.	Regional	v.	Brachiocephalic
c.	Arteriole	m.	Venule	w.	Common
d.	Venous	n.	Vascular	x.	Three
e.	Deep	o.	Superficial	y.	Lymphatic
f.	Capillary	p.	Externa	z.	Vein
g.	Valves	q.	Tunica		
h.	Anastomosis	r.	Blood		
i.	Sinuses	s.	Vascular plexus		
j.	Intima	t.	Media		

1. Large network of blood vessels _____

2. Communication mode for blood vessels by connecting channels _____

3. Layers noted in blood vessels _____

4. Outer connective tissue layer in blood vessels _____

5. Middle smooth muscle layer with varying elastic fibers _____

6. Inner endothelium that lines the blood vessels _____

7. Arises from the heart and carries blood away _____

8. Blood supply that has arteries _____

9. Smaller-diameter artery _____

10. Smaller diameter than an arteriole

11. Smaller diameter than vein _____

12. Drainage of blood _____

13. Blood vessel that travels to the heart carrying blood to it _____

14. Vein property preventing blood from flowing backward _____

15. Blood-filled spaces between two layers of tissue _____

16. Less numerous than lymphatic vessels _____

17. Pathway mainly parallels blood vessels _____

18. Veins that are found immediately deep to skin _____

19. Veins that usually accompany larger arteries _____

20. Number of classes for both arteries and veins _____

21. System of arterial blood supply, capillary network, and venous drainage _____

22. Present with capillaries for exchange of oxygen and carbon dioxide _____

23. Property of the blood supply as to coverage _____

24. Common carotid and subclavian arteries arise from it on left side _____

25. Direct branch of the aorta _____

26. Carotid that travels superiorly branchless along neck _____

True or False

Assign the statement below as either true or false. For deeper understanding, edit the false statements until they are true.

1. Both the head and neck contain certain important venous plexuses. _____

2. Blood vessels communicate with each other. _____

3. Three layers are in differing amounts for an artery, a capillary, and a vein. _____

4. Each artery starts out as a small-diameter vessels. _____

5. Veins branch into smaller diameter vessels becoming a capillary network. _____

6. Each capillary can supply blood to a larger area due to increased numbers. _____

7. Most veins of the face, but not all, have valves. _____

8. Veins pump blood at higher pressures, which naturally prevents backflow. _____

9. Dental professionals need to understand the structure of the heart. _____

10. Unlike nerves, blood vessels have a one-to-one relationship to structures. _____

11. The common carotid artery travels in the carotid sheath deep to the SCM. _____

12. The external and internal carotids lie side by side within the carotid triangle. _____

13. Carotid sinus is a swelling that can be palpated against the thyroid gland. _____

14. Carotid pulse is the most reliable pulse. _____

15. Subclavian artery arises lateral to the common carotid artery. _____

16. Internal carotid artery travels slightly lateral to external carotid artery. _____

17. Internal carotid artery is covered in the neck by the large masseter muscle. _____

18. External carotid artery supplies the oral cavity. _____

19. The external carotid artery has five sets of branches. _____

20. The only medial branch from external carotid artery. _____

21. Branches of external carotid artery are the occipital and posterior auricular. _____

22. Terminal branches of external carotid artery are the temporal and aorta. _____

23. Maxillary artery is the largest terminal branch of the external carotid artery. _____

24. Maxillary artery courses between the muscles of mastication. _____

25. Maxillary artery has three parts designated by location. _____

26. The maxillary artery has a standard set course and branching patterns. _____

27. One side branching of the maxillary artery predicts the contralateral side. _____

28. The first part of the maxillary artery is also considered the mandibular part. _____

29. Maxillary artery's second part enters the pterygopalatine fossa. _____

30. Third part of the maxillary artery is associated with pterygopalatine fossa. _____

Charting

Fill in the rest of the flowchart from the indicated textbook figure.
Figure 6.4: Branches of the external carotid artery.

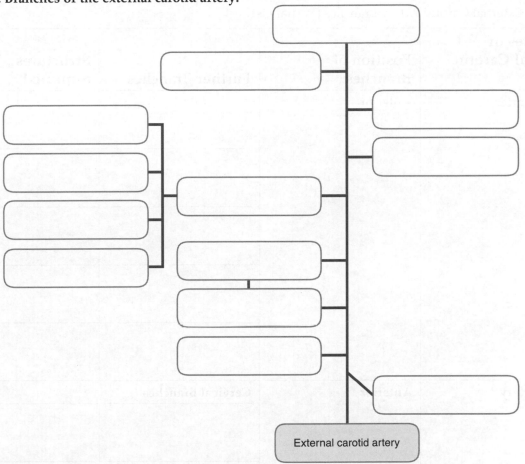

External carotid artery

Figure 6.10: Branches of the maxillary artery.

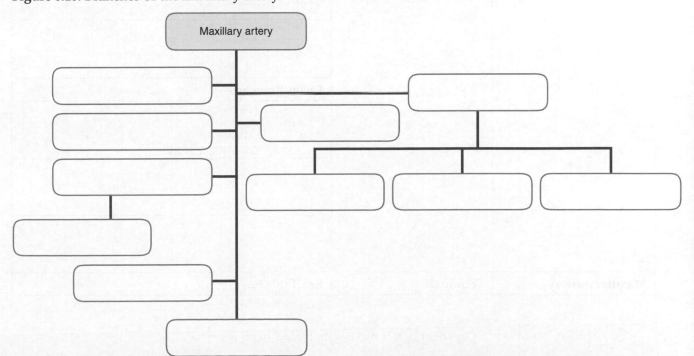

Maxillary artery

Table Completion

Fill in the rest of the table from the indicated textbook table.

Table 6.1 External Carotid Artery Branches (Partial List)

Branches of External Carotid Artery	Position of Branches	Further Branches	Structures Supplied
Lingual artery	Anterior		
Facial artery	Anterior	Cervical Branches	
		Facial Branches	
Maxillary artery	Terminal	See Table 6.2.	

Table 6.2 Maxillary Artery Branches (Partial List)

Major Branches of Maxillary Artery With Part Noted	Further Branches	Structures Supplied
First Part		
Inferior alveolar artery		
Second Part		
Buccal artery		
Third Part		
Posterior superior alveolar artery		
Infraorbital artery		
	Middle superior alveolar artery, if present	
Descending palatine artery		
Sphenopalatine artery		

Table 6.3 Veins of the Head (Partial List)

Region or Tributaries Drained	Drainage Veins	Major Veins/Sinuses
Upper lip area		
Maxillary teeth with periodontium and gingiva		
Lower lip area		
Mandibular teeth with periodontium and gingiva and submental region		
Submental region		
Lingual and sublingual regions		
Deep facial areas and posterior superior alveolar and inferior alveolar veins		
Pterygoid plexus of veins		

CHAPTER 7: GLANDULAR TISSUE

Note: Answers can be obtained from your instructor and their Evolve Resources unless from textbook source.

Matching

Match each item below with its best short description; each single item can only be matched once.

a.	Lacrimal	k.	Maxillary second	u.	Masseter
b.	Xerostomia	l.	Parotidectomy	v.	Submandibular
c.	Conjunctiva	m.	Mumps	w.	Parotid
d.	Facial	n.	Parotitis	x.	Major
e.	Minor	o.	Thyroid	y.	Thyroxine
f.	Dry eye	p.	Lingual	z.	Posterior cheek
g.	Saliva	q.	Hyposalivation		
h.	Motor	r.	Sublingual		
i.	Endocrine	s.	Gland		
j.	Exocrine	t.	Glandular		

1. Lacrimal, salivary, thyroid, parathyroid, and thymus _____

2. Producing chemical secretion necessary for body functioning _____

3. Type of gland that has an associated duct _____

4. Gland that does not have a duct but empties directly _____

5. Nerves that regulate the flow of secretions from glands _____

6. Paired almond-shaped glands that secrete lacrimal fluid _____

7. Lacrimal fluid lubricates this part of the eyes _____

8. Syndrome of the eyes that can accompany dry mouth _____

9. Secretion produced by the salivary glands _____

10. Large paired salivary glands with named ducts _____

11. Largest encapsulated major salivary gland _____

12. Nerve divides parotid salivary gland into two lobes _____

13. Muscle that the parotid gland mostly overlies _____

14. Parotid duct is on the inner buccal mucosa opposite this molar _____

15. Inflammatory enlargement of parotid salivary gland _____

16. Viral infection of parotid salivary gland _____

17. Parotid gland cancer location in most cases _____

18. Surgical removal of parotid salivary gland _____

19. Hook-shaped gland that has two lobes _____

20. Gland anterior to submandibular gland _____

21. Nerve located near submandibular duct _____

22. Type of salivary gland more numerous and without capsules _____

23. Reduced production of saliva _____

24. Dry mouth associated with DES _____

25. Largest endocrine gland _____

26. Thyroid gland secretion without ducts _____

True or False

Assign the statement below as either true or false. For deeper understanding, edit the false statements until they are true.

1. Lacrimal gland has palpebral and orbital parts. _____

2. The nasolacrimal duct begins in the temporal fossa and passes superiorly. _____

3. Tears collect and then pass over the eye surface to the lacrimal punctum. _____

4. Any lacrimal fluid that passes over the eye ends up in the lacrimal sac. _____

5. Saliva only lubricates the oral cavity and has no other function. _____

6. Functioning of salivary ducts are noted during an extraoral examination. _____

7. Parotid papilla is a small elevation of tissue that marks the parotid duct. _____

8. Most salivary gland cancers involve the parotid salivary gland. _____

9. Parotid can be pierced by IA block traumatizing the facial nerve. _____

10. Submandibular salivary gland is the main contributor to salivary volume. _____

11. Sublingual salivary gland is the most commonly involved with stones. _____

12. The ducts of Rivinus open along the oral vestibules. _____

13. Minor salivary glands are not found in the gingival tissue. _____

14. Most minor salivary glands secrete mainly a mucous type of product. _____

15. Salivary stones can cause gland enlargement and tenderness. _____

16. Certain medications or diseases can cause hyposalivation. _____

17. Xerostomia can be associated with DES, since they have similar causes. _____

18. Salivary replacements can help xerostomia. _____

19. Thyroxine depresses the metabolic rate of the body. _____

20. In a healthy patient, the thyroid gland is not visible. _____

21. An enlarged thyroid gland is considered a goiter. _____

22. An enlarged thyroid gland may be firm and tender with masses. _____

23. A diseased thyroid gland never loses its mobility. _____

24. Usually the thyroid gland moves upward when swallowing. _____

25. Diseased parathyroid glands may alter the thyroid gland function. _____

26. Parathyroid glands help regulate calcium and phosphorus levels. _____

27. The thymus gland is also part of the immune system. _____

28. The B-cell lymphocytes mature within the thymus gland. _____

29. After puberty, the thymus gland undergoes involution. _____

30. The thymus gland is considered a temporary structure. _____

Table Completion

Fill in the rest of the table from the indicated textbook table.

Table 7.1 Head and Neck Glands

Gland	Location	Associated Innervation	Lymphatic Drainage	Blood Supply
Lacrimal gland with lacrimal ducts				
Parotid salivary gland with parotid duct				
Submandibular salivary gland with submandibular duct				
Sublingual salivary gland with ducts of Rivinus and/or sublingual duct(s)				
Minor salivary glands with ducts				
Thyroid gland				
Parathyroid glands				
Thymus gland				

CHAPTER 8: NERVOUS SYSTEM

Note: Answers can be obtained from your instructor and their Evolve Resources unless from textbook source.

Matching

Match each item below with its best short description; each single item can only be matched once.

a.	Innervation	k.	Anesthesia	u.	Cerebrospinal fluid
b.	Spinal cord	l.	Brain	v.	Pia mater
c.	Dura mater	m.	Ganglion	w.	Subarachnoid mater
d.	Meninges	n.	Core bundles	x.	Fascicles
c.	Afferent	o.	Mantle bundles	y.	Arachnoid mater
f.	Efferent	p.	Paresthesia	z.	Nervous system
g.	Proprioception	q.	Central		
h.	Neuron	r.	Peripheral		
i.	Neurotransmitter	s.	Muscles		
j.	Nerve	t.	Synapse		

1. Extensive and intricate network of neural structures _____

2. Nervous system causes these to contract for joint movements _____

3. Nervous system has the CNS and this other division _____

4. Cellular component of nervous system _____

5. Bundle of neural processes outside the CNS and in the PNS _____

6. Junction between two neurons or neuron and infector organ _____

7. Supply of nerves to body part _____

8. Accumulation of neuron cell bodies outside the CNS _____

9. Bundles of nerves _____

10. Fascicles within the innermost of nerve _____

11. Fascicles near outer surface of nerve. _____

12. Sensory nerve carrying information to brain _____

13. Motor nerve carrying information from brain _____

14. Information concerning body movement and position _____

15. Chemical agent for impulse to cross the synapse _____

16. Loss of feeling or sensation _____

17. Abnormal sensation involving trauma or toxicity _____

18. Major division of nervous system _____

19. Membranes of the brain _____

20. Meninges layer that also surrounds and supports the dural sinuses _____

21. Middle layer of meninges _____

22. Underneath arachnoid mater _____

23 Innermost layer of meninges _____

24. Fluid within subarachnoid mater _____

25. The CNS includes the brain and this structure _____

26. Has major divisions of cerebrum, cerebellum, brainstem, diencephalon _____

True or False

Assign the statement below as either true or false. For deeper understanding, edit the false statements until they are true.

1. The largest division of the brain is the cerebellum. _____

2. The cerebrum consists of two cerebral hemispheres. _____

3. The brainstem includes the medulla, pons, and midbrain. _____

4. Cell bodies of fifth and seventh cranial nerves are in the pons. _____

5. The diencephalon includes the midbrain. _____

6. The thalamus regulates body temperature and blood pressure. _____

7. The spinal cord has both gray and white matter. _____

8. Some spinal cord tracts ascend and others descend to the brain. _____

9. The PNS is further divided into the afferent and efferent nervous systems. _____

10. The SNS includes only efferent nerves. _____

11. The ANS acts without any conscious control. _____

12. The parasympathetic system is involved in aiding digestion. _____

13. The cranial nerves are an important part of the PNS. _____

14. The ten paired cranial nerves are connected to the brain at its base. _____

15. All cranial nerves are efferent in their neural processes. _____

16. Olfactory (first cranial) nerve enters the skull through the cribriform plate. _____

17. Optic (second cranial) nerves join at the optic chiasma. _____

18. Oculomotor (third cranial) nerve is an efferent nerve to eye muscles._____

19. Trochlear (fourth cranial) nerve first runs up the lateral wall of orbit. _____

20. Trigeminal (fifth cranial) nerve has both efferent and afferent components. _____

21. The trigeminal nerve is the largest cranial nerve. _____

22. The trigeminal nerve has two nerve divisions. _____

23. Maxillary nerve enters the skull via the foramen ovale. _____

24. Mandibular nerve enters the skull via the foramen rotundum. _____

25. Abducens (sixth cranial) nerve exits the skull via superior orbital fissure. _____

26. Facial (seventh cranial) nerve has only afferent components. _____

27. The eighth cranial nerve carries efferent for muscles of facial expression. _____

28. The ninth cranial nerve passes through the skull via the jugular foramen. _____

29. Otic ganglion is located near the foramen ovale. _____

30. Vagus (tenth cranial) nerve caries components to many organs. _____

31. The eleventh cranial nerve functions for the trapezius and SCM muscles._____

32. The twelfth cranial nerve serves the intrinsic and extrinsic tongue muscles. _____

33. Trigeminal ganglion is a bulge in the sensory root of the trigeminal nerve. _____

34. First division of the trigeminal nerve travels via the superior orbital fissure. _____

35. Maxillary nerve is a nerve trunk formed within the pterygopalatine fossa. _____

36. The pterygopalatine ganglion serves fibers from facial nerve. _____

37. Zygomatic nerve enters pterygopalatine fossa via superior orbital fissure. _____

38. Infraorbital nerve passes into the infraorbital foramen of the maxilla. _____

39. A dental plexus is a network of nerves within both dental arches. _____

40. Crossover-innervation is overlap of contralateral terminal nerve fibers. _____

41. The MSA nerve is present in over 75% of the population. _____

42. The PSA nerve joins the IO nerve within the pterygopalatine fossa. _____

43. Patients may gag when there is anesthesia of the LP nerve. _____

44. Both the right and left NP nerves enter the greater palatine foramen. _____

45. The (long) buccal is initially located on the buccinator muscle. _____

46 Lingual nerve communicates with the submandibular ganglion. _____

47. The IA nerve is formed from merger of mental and incisive nerves. _____

48. The IA nerve exits the mandible via the mental foramen. _____

49. Mental foramen is usually inferior to apices of mandibular canines. _____

50. Both the mental and lingual foramina can be noted radiographically. _____

Charting

Fill in the rest of the flowchart from the indicated textbook figure.
Figure 8.2: Divisions of the nervous system.

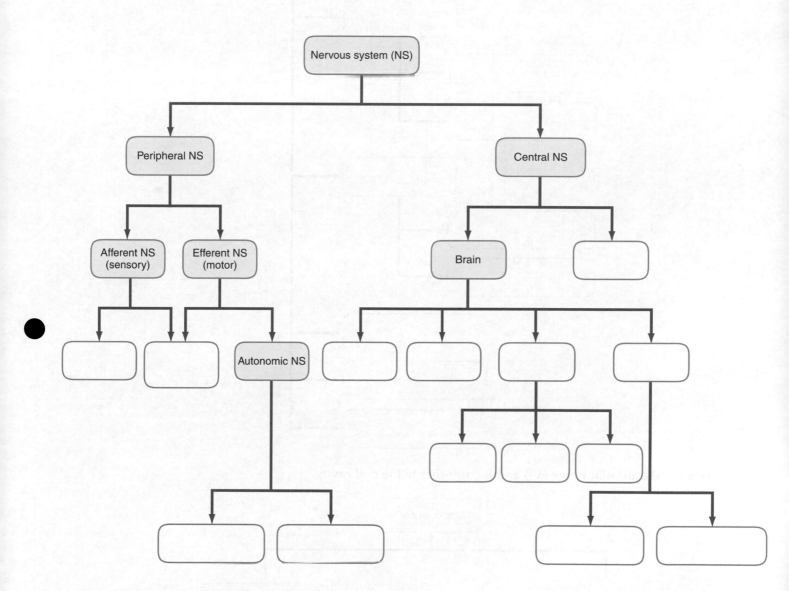

Figure 8.12: Maxillary nerve (V₂) and its branches to the oral cavity.

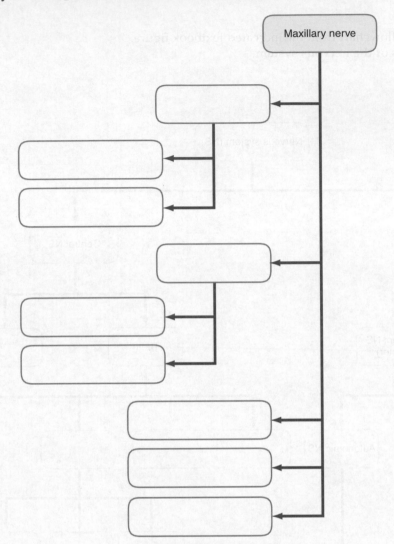

Figure 8.17: Mandibular nerve (V₃) and its branches to the oral cavity.

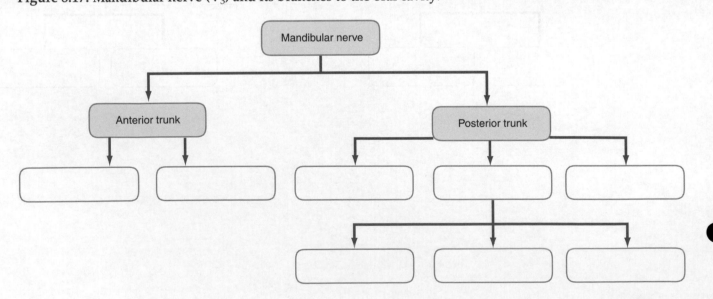

Table Completion

Fill in the rest of the table from the indicated textbook table.

Table 8.1 Cranial Nerve Innervations

Nerve (Roman Numeral/Name)		Nerve Types: Structures Innervated
I		Afferent:
II		Afferent:
III		Efferent:
IV		Efferent:
V		Efferent:
		Afferent:
VI		Efferent:
VII		Efferent:
		Afferent:
VIII		Afferent:
IX		Efferent:
		Afferent:

Continued

Table 8.1 Cranial Nerve Innervations—cont'd

Nerve (Roman Numeral/Name)		Nerve Types: Structures Innervated
X		Efferent:
		Afferent:
XI		Efferent:
XII		Efferent:

Table 8.2 Orofacial Structures Innervation

Orofacial Structures	Nerves: Fiber Type
Maxillary anterior teeth and associated labial periodontium and gingiva	
Maxillary posterior teeth and associated buccal periodontium and gingiva as well as maxillary sinus	
Anterior hard palate and associated palatal periodontium and gingiva of maxillary anterior teeth as well as nasal septum	
Posterior hard palate and associated palatal periodontium and gingiva of maxillary posterior teeth	
Soft palate and palatine tonsils	
Mandibular teeth and associated facial periodontium and gingiva of mandibular anterior teeth and premolars as well as labial mucosa	

Table 8.2 Orofacial Structures Innervation—cont'd

Orofacial Structures	Nerves: Fiber Type
Associated buccal periodontium and gingiva of mandibular molars as well as buccal mucosa	
Associated lingual periodontium and gingiva of mandibular teeth as well as floor of mouth	
Tongue—general sensation	
Tongue—taste sensation	
Tongue muscles	
Parotid salivary gland	
Submandibular and sublingual salivary glands	
Lacrimal gland	
Muscles of facial expression	
Muscles of mastication	
Trapezius and sternocleidomastoid muscles	

CHAPTER 9: ANATOMY OF LOCAL ANESTHESIA

Note: Answers can be obtained from your instructor and their Evolve Resources unless from textbook source.

Matching

Match each item below with its best short description; each single item can only be matched once.

a.	Nerve block	k.	Mandible	u.	Crossover
b.	Abscess	l.	Facial paralysis	v.	Blanch
c.	Maxillae	m.	Mucobuccal	w.	Shock
d.	Parotid salivary	n.	Core	x.	Mesiobuccal
e.	Density	o.	Positive aspiration	y.	Pterygomandibular
f.	Panoramic	p.	Soreness	z.	Supraperiosteal injection
g.	Hard tissue	q.	Swallowing		
h.	Anatomic variation	r.	Pressure anesthesia		
i.	Sphenomandibular	s.	Middle		
j.	Mantle	t.	Lingual		

1. Smaller area for anesthesia in the oral cavity _____

2. Local anesthesia of a larger area _____

3. Its presence precludes any anesthesia _____

4. More clinically effective with local anesthesia than that of mandible _____

5. Mandible is less clinically effective due to this reason _____

6. Maxillae has less of this than the mandible _____

7. More troubleshooting with lack of clinical effectiveness than maxillae _____

8. Superior alveolar nerve that is not always present _____

9. Maxillary first molar root not always innervated by PSA nerve _____

10. PSA block has needle inserted into the height of this fold _____

11. PSA block has a high risk of this occurring even correctly given _____

12. Occurrence with pressure applied to infraorbital foramen _____

13. Its use reduces patient discomfort with both NP and GP blocks _____

14. What occurs with pressure anesthesia to tissue _____

15. IA block anesthetizes not only the IA nerve but also this nerve _____

16. Bundles that innervate the posterior mandible _____

17. Bundles that innervate the anterior mandible _____

18 Bilateral IA blocks can cause difficulty with this _____

19. Type of landmarks mainly used during IA block _____

20. Pterygomandibular fold overlies this raphe _____

21. Radiograph that helps with troubleshooting the IA block _____

22. Ligament that can act as barrier with IA block _____

23. Feeling as needle passes by the lingual nerve _____

24. Transient complication with IA block due to piercing gland _____

25. Gland that carries terminal branches of facial nerve _____

26. Type of innervation that can be reduced with incisive nerve block _____

True or False

Assign the statement below as either true or false. For deeper understanding, edit the false statements until they are true.

1. A MSA block is recommended after the PSA block. _____

2. Foramina for PSA block are posterosuperior to maxillary tuberosity. _____

3. The maxilla is contacted during the PSA block to reduce trauma. _____

4. Syringe barrel extends from contralateral labial commissure for PSA block. _____

5. Gently tapping on the molar teeth is recommended for PSA block. _____

6. Harmless anesthesia of mandibular nerve can occur with PSA block. _____

7. An extraoral hematoma is a risk with the PSA block. _____

8. If using contaminated needle with PSA block, spread of infection can occur. _____

9. The MSA nerve is part of the superior dental plexus. _____

10. The MSA block has a high risk of positive aspiration and overinsertion. _____

11. The ASA block is commonly used with MSA block instead of IO block. _____

12. The ASA nerve has crossover-innervation in many cases. _____

13. The IO block covers the regions covered by the MSA and ASA nerves. _____

14. The NP and GP blocks may be used for complete coverage after IO block. _____

15. The IO foramen is only intraorally palpated before the IO block. _____

16. There is a linear relationship of IO foramen and the mental symphysis. _____

17. The finger of the other hand is always on the IO foramen during IO block. _____

18. Maintaining contact with the bone during IO block reduces complications. _____

19. Pressure anesthesia for GP block produces a dull ache to block pain. _____

20. The LP foramen must be palpated before the GP block is given. _____

21. The GP foramen will appear closer to dentition with more shallow palate. _____

22. Soft palate may become uncomfortably anesthetized with GP block. _____

23. Pressure anesthesia is used on the contralateral side of incisive papilla. _____

24. Incisive foramen is at midline between palatine processes of maxillae. _____

25. The needle cannot enter incisive foramen using recommended positions. _____

26. The IA block is considered by anatomists to be a *true* mandibular block. _____

27. Core bundles of anterior mandibular teeth take time to anesthetize. _____

28. Additional use of buccal block may be indicated after the IA block. _____

29. Crossover-innervation may present with the lingual nerve. _____

30. Agent must be placed within at least 10 mm of target area with IA block. _____

31. Hard tissue landmarks are mainly used for IA block to reduce errors. _____

32. Pterygomandibular fold become accentuated with opening the mouth. _____

33. With IA block, the mandibular ramus can be extraorally palpated. _____

34. The buccal fat pad or tongue may create problems with IA block. _____

35. Not necessary to deposit small amounts of agent during IA block. _____

36. It may be necessary to reinject a patient with IA block. _____

37. Medial surface of mandibular ramus is contacted during IA block. _____

38. Lingual nerve may be inadvertently contacted during IA block. _____

39. The syringe barrel is parallel to the occlusal plane with buccal block. _____

40. Self-inflicted trauma never occurs after a buccal block. _____

41. The mental foramen can be located on a radiograph. _____

42. The mental foramen in adults faces posterosuperiorly. _____

43. The needle always enters the mental foramen with mental block._____

44. The mental block has a high risk of positive aspiration. _____

45. Pressure on mental foramen causes soreness due to nearby nerve. _____

46. More agent is used with the incisive block than mental block. _____

47. Soft tissue anesthesia proceeds pulpal with incisive block. _____

48. Harmless tingling of lower lip occurs with incisive block. _____

49. Pressure is applied to injection site with incisive block. _____

50. Incisive block is used for crossover-innervation in maxillae. _____

Table Completion

Fill in the rest of the table from the indicated textbook table.

Table 9.3 Review of Local Anesthesia of the Dentition and Related Structures

Maxillary Anesthesia			
Structures Anesthetized	**Landmarks**	**Target Area**	**Injection Site**
PSA Block			
Nerves: Teeth: Other Structures:			
MSA Block			
Nerves: Teeth: Other Structures:			
ASA Block			
Nerves: Teeth: Other Structures:			

Table 9.3 Review of Local Anesthesia of the Dentition and Related Structures—cont'd

Maxillary Anesthesia			
Structures Anesthetized	**Landmarks**	**Target Area**	**Injection Site**
IO Block			
Nerves: Teeth: Other Structures:	Extraoral: Intraoral:		
GP Block			
Nerves: Teeth: Other Structures:			
NP Block			
Nerves: Teeth: Other Structures:			

Continued

Table 9.3 Review of Local Anesthesia of the Dentition and Related Structures—cont'd

Maxillary Anesthesia			
Structures Anesthetized	**Landmarks**	**Target Area**	**Injection Site**
AMSA Block			
Nerves: Teeth: Other Structures:			
Mandibular Anesthesia			
IA Block			
Nerves: Teeth: Other Structures:			
Buccal Block			
Nerves: Teeth: Other Structures:			

Table 9.3 Review of Local Anesthesia of the Dentition and Related Structures—cont'd

Mandibular Anesthesia			
Structures Anesthetized	**Landmarks**	**Target Area**	**Injection Site**
Mental Block			
Nerves: **Teeth:** **Other Structures:**			
Incisive Block			
Nerves: **Teeth:** **Other Structures:**			

Continued

Table 9.3 Review of Local Anesthesia of the Dentition and Related Structures—cont'd

Mandibular Anesthesia			
Structures Anesthetized	**Landmarks**	**Target Area**	**Injection Site**
Gow-Gates Mandibular Block			
Nerves: **Teeth:** **Other Structures:**	**Extraoral:** **Intraoral:**		
Vazirani-Akinosi Mandibular Block			
Nerves: **Teeth:** **Other Structures:**			

CHAPTER 10: LYMPHATIC SYSTEM

Note: Answers can be obtained from your instructor and their Evolve Resources unless from textbook source.

Matching

Match each item below with its best short description; each single item can only be matched once.

a.	Secondary	k.	Backflow	u.	Generalized
b.	Lymph	l.	Lymphadenopathy	v.	Airways
c.	Afferent vessels	m.	Glands	w.	Tonsils
d.	Venous drainage	n.	Efferent vessel	x.	Lymph nodes
e.	Spread	o.	Lymphatic ducts	y.	Medical referral
f.	Jugular trunk	p.	Primary	z.	Lymphocytes
g.	Right lymphatic duct	q.	Tender		
h.	Hilus	r.	One-way valves		
i.	Thoracic duct	s.	Lymphatic vessels		
j.	Lymphadenitis	t.	Lymphatic system		

1. Consisting of vessels, nodes, ducts, and tonsils _____

2. Channels that parallel the venous blood vessels _____

3. Tissue fluid draining from surrounding region into lymphatic vessels _____

4. What lymphatic vessels have that capillaries do not _____

5. Bean-shaped bodies along lymphatic vessels _____

6. What lymph nodes are called by patients _____

7. Lymph nodes are involved in this production _____

8. Lymph flowing into lymph node _____

9. Lymph flowing out of lymph node _____

10. Depression associated with the efferent vessel _____

11. Type of node where lymph drains from first _____

12. Type of node where lymph drains into from primary node _____

13. Masses of lymphoid tissue _____

14. Where tonsils are located along with food passages _____

15. Lymph vessels converge into larger structures _____

16. Where lymphatic ducts empty into _____

17. Lymphatic system of right side by way of this _____

18. At junction of the right subclavian and right internal jugular veins _____

19. From left jugular trunk into this _____

20. One-way valves on lymphatic duct prevent this _____

21. Dramatic increase in lymph node size and consistency _____

22. When more than one group of nodes is enlarged _____

23. Lymph nodes undergoing inflammation _____

24. How nodes with lymphadenopathy can feel when palpated _____

25. Needed when patient has palpable nodes associated with disease _____

26. This can occur along connecting lymphatic vessels with infection _____

True or False

Assign the statement below as either true or false. For deeper understanding, edit the false statements until they are true.

1. Nodes can be superficially located or located deep. _____

2. Nodes in healthy patient cannot be visualized or felt when palpating. _____

3. Lymphatic system fights disease processes such as infection and cancer. _____

4. Lymphatic vessels are less numerous than venous blood vessels. _____

5. Lymph is a thick viscous fluid. _____

6. Lymphatic vessels are smaller and thinner than capillaries. _____

7. Nodes are positioned beside lymphatic vessels so as to filter toxins. _____

8. In health, nodes are small, soft, and mobile in surrounding tissue. _____

9. Node drainage goes from deep to superficial placement. _____

10. Tonsils contain lymphocytes that remove toxins. _____

11. Thoracic duct is much larger than right lymphatic duct. _____

12 Lymph nodes are paired and drain either right or left tissue. _____

13. Left lymphatic duct drains entire lower half of the body. _____

14. Final drainage endpoint of lymphatic vessels mirrors vascular system. _____

15. Lymphadenopathy can also occur to the tonsils. _____

16. Lymphadenopathy is from larger lymphocytes and increased numbers. _____

17. Lymphadenopathy allows the nodes to be visualized and palpated. _____

18. Palpation of nodes is against backdrop of the soft tissue areas. _____

19. Nodes must be larger than about 5 mm to be seen and felt. _____

20. Palpable lymph nodes need to be recorded in patient's chart. _____

Charting

Fill in the rest of the flowchart from the indicated textbook figure.
Figure 10.8: Lymphatic drainage of the head into the neck.

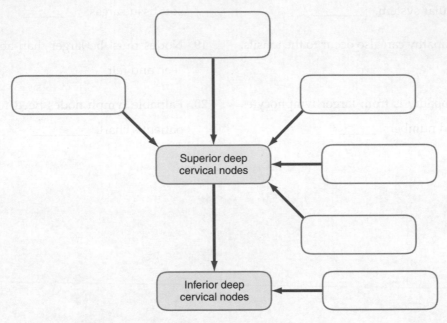

Figure 10.11: Superficial lymphatic drainage of the neck.

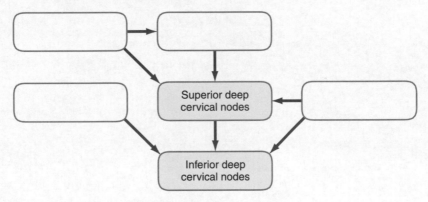

Figure 10.16: Lymphatic drainage of the neck.

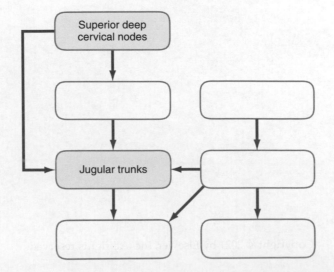

Table Completion

Fill in the rest of the table from the indicated textbook table

Table 10.1 Oral Cavity Lymph Node Drainage

Structures	Primary Nodes	Secondary Nodes
Buccal mucosa		
Anterior hard palate		
Posterior hard palate		
Soft palate		
Maxillary anterior teeth with periodontium and gingiva		
Maxillary first and second molars and premolars with periodontium and gingiva		
Maxillary third molars with periodontium and gingiva		
Mandibular incisors with periodontium and gingiva		
Mandibular canines, premolars, and molars with periodontium and gingiva		

Continued

Table 10.1 Oral Cavity Lymph Node Drainage—cont'd

Structures	Primary Nodes	Secondary Nodes
Floor of the mouth		
Apex of the tongue		
Body of the tongue		
Base of the tongue		
Palatine tonsils and lingual tonsil		

Table 10.2 Head and Face Lymph Node Drainage (Partial List)

Structures	Primary Nodes	Secondary Nodes
External ear		
Middle ear		
Paranasal sinuses		
Infraorbital region and nasal cavity		
Cheek in buccal region		
Upper lip		
Lower lip		

Table 10.3 Cervical Lymph Node Drainage

Structures	Primary Nodes	Secondary Nodes
Superficial anterior cervical triangle		
Superficial lateral and posterior cervical triangles		
Deep posterior cervical triangle		
Pharynx		
Thyroid gland		
Larynx		
Esophagus		
Trachea		

CHAPTER 11: FASCIAE AND SPACES

Note: Answers can be obtained from your instructor and their Evolve Resources unless from textbook source.

Matching

Match each item below with its best short description; each single item can only be matched once.

a.	Skin	k.	Vertebral	u.	Visceral
b.	Platysma	l.	Infection	v.	Bones
c.	Fascial spaces	m.	Superficial cervical	w.	Buccopharyngeal
d.	Sheetlike	n.	Tenth (vagus)	x.	Investing
e.	Carotid sheath	o.	Pterygoid	y.	Submental
f.	Masticator	p.	Inelastic	z.	Sublingual
g.	Buccal	q.	Infratemporal		
h.	Canine	r.	Fascia		
i.	Submandibular	s.	Blood vessels		
j.	Superficial facial	t.	Jaws		

1. Layers upon layers of fibrous connective tissue _____

2. Lies above deeper fascia along with the muscles, bones, nerves, organs _____

3. Potential spaces created between layers of fascia _____

4. Nature of fascia _____

5. What travels along in the superficial fasciae of the body besides nerves _____

6. Fascia of face enclosed by most of the muscles of facial expression _____

7. Muscle within superficial cervical fascia of the neck _____

8. Continuous with the layers of deep fascia of the face _____

9. Deep cervical fasciae is more complex than this fascia _____

10. Layers of deep fascia consist of this dense fibrous tissue _____

11. The most external layer of deep cervical fascia _____

12. Bilateral tube of deep cervical fascia deep to SCM muscle _____

13. The carotid sheath contains this cranial nerve _____

14. Fascia that encloses the entire superior part of alimentary canal _____

15. Fascia that covers the floor of the anterior cervical triangle _____

16. Fascia that covers spinal cord and cervical vertebrae _____

17. Communication with fascial spaces allows the spread of this _____

18. Fascial spaces are defined by arrangement of muscles and these _____

19. Space superior to upper lip _____

20. Space formed between buccinator muscle and masseter muscle _____

21. Space of entire area of mandible and muscles of mastication _____

22. Space that occupies the infratemporal fossa _____

23. Infratemporal space contains this plexus of veins _____

24. Space located between mandibular symphysis and hyoid bone _____

25. Cross-sectional shape of bilateral space is triangular _____

26. Floor of this space is the mylohyoid muscle _____

True or False

Assign the statement below as either true or false. For deeper understanding, edit the false statements until they are true.

1. Fascial spaces are really empty spaces. _____

2. Other structures can create spaces such as bones and muscles. _____

3. Fascia and resulting spaces study helps understand anatomic regions. _____

4. Layers of superficial fascia can vary in thickness. _____

5. Temporal fascia covers structures superior to zygomatic arch. _____

6. Investing fascia splits around three salivary glands. _____

7. The visceral fascia is deep and parallel to the carotid sheath. _____

8. Posterior and lateral to pharynx is the buccopharyngeal fascia. _____

9. A dental infection in canine space leads nasolabial sulcus loss of depth. _____

10. A dental infection with buccal space leads to a swollen cheek. _____

11. Infratemporal space contains part of the maxillary artery and its branches. _____

12. Source of infratemporal space infection is usually mandibular third molar. _____

13. Pterygomandibular space has the mandibular ramus as its lateral wall. _____

14. Source of pterygomandibular space infection is mainly mandibular molars. _____

15. Severe trismus is possibly with infection in pterygomandibular space. _____

16. An infection in the submasseteric space can involve pericoronitis. _____

17. Infection of space of body of mandible appears as enlarged mandible. _____

18. Submental space coincides with the submandibular triangle. _____

19. Submandibular space infection may lead to Ludwig angina. _____

20. Parapharyngeal space is a single tube lateral to medial pterygoid muscle. _____

21. Retropharyngeal space is a danger risk by healthcare professionals. _____

22. Dental infections in retropharyngeal space can lead to airway obstruction. _____

23. Vertebral compartment contains the spinal cord and cervical vertebrae. _____

24. Bilateral visceral compartment contains the orbit and its contents. _____

25. Vascular compartments consist of two carotid sheaths. _____

Table Completion

Fill in the rest of the table from the indicated textbook table

Table 11.1 Fasciae of Head and Neck

Fasciae of Head and Neck	Relationship to Head and Neck Structures
Superficial Fasciae of Face and Neck	
Superficial fascia of face	
Superficial cervical fascia of neck	
Deep Fasciae of Face and Jaws (Continuous With Investing Layer of Deep Cervical Fascia as Well as Each Other)	
Temporal fascia	
Masseteric-parotid fascia	
Pterygoid fascia	
Deep Cervical Fasciae (From External to Internal in Location and Continuous With Each Other)	
Investing fascia	
Carotid sheath	
Visceral fascia	
Buccopharyngeal fascia	
Vertebral fascia	

Table 11.2 Major Spaces of Face and Jaws (Partial List)

Space	Location	Contents	Communication Pattern	Source of Possible Infection
Canine space				
Buccal space				
Parotid space				
Temporal space				
Infratemporal space				
Pterygomandibular space				
Submasseteric space				
Submental space				
Submandibular space				
Sublingual space				

Table 11.3 Major Cervical Fascial Spaces

Space	Location	Contents	Communication Pattern
Previsceral			
Parapharyngeal			

Table 11.3 Major Cervical Fascial Spaces—cont'd

Space	Location	Contents	Communication Pattern
Retropharyngeal			
Perivertebral			

Table 11.4 Cervical Compartments With Contents and Borders

Cervical Compartment	Contents	Border
Vertebral compartment		
Visceral compartment		
Vascular compartments		

CHAPTER 12: SPREAD OF INFECTION

Note: Answers can be obtained from your instructor and their Evolve Resources unless from textbook source.

Matching

Match each item below with its best short description; each single item can only be matched once.

a.	Microbiota	k.	Pustule	u.	Necrosis
b.	Odontogenic	l.	Cellulitis	v.	Bacteremia
c.	Beta-lactamases	m.	Involucrum	w.	Cavernous sinus thrombosis
d.	Abscess	n.	Opportunistic	x.	Cephalosporin
e.	Periapical	o.	Upper respiratory	y.	Suppuration
f.	Pathogens	p.	Pericoronal	z.	Periodontal
g.	Pericoronitis	q.	Osteomyelitis		
h.	Stoma	r.	Fistula		
i.	Surgical drainage	s.	Sequestrum		
j.	Virulence	t.	Resident		

1. Regional collection or community of microbes _____

2. Indigenous type of microbiota in a healthy body _____

3. Nonresident microorganisms that can invade and initiate an infection _____

4. Factors that help pathogens further the infection process _____

5. Infection that involves the teeth or associated tissue _____

6. Enzymes produced by gram-negative anaerobic bacteria _____

7. Class C beta-lactamases result in this antibiotic resistance _____

8. Localized entrapment of pathogens in closed space _____

9. Type of abscess that is most common odontogenic emergency _____

10. Less common type of odontogenic emergency abscess type _____

11. Least common type of odontogenic emergency abscess type _____

12. Further formation of tracts with chronic abscess formation _____

13. Pus that contains pathogenic bacteria _____

14. Another name given to *pericoronal abscess* _____

15. With odontogenic infections, the overlying tissue undergoes this _____

16. Small elevated lesion of either skin or oral mucosa _____

17. Opening of the fistula from the tract _____

18. Most common treatment for suppurating odontogenic infections _____

19. Diffuse inflammation of soft tissue spaces _____

20. Inflammation of bone marrow _____

21. Devitalized bone surrounded by infected exudate _____

22. New bone among the sequestrum _____

23. An infection when the body's innate defenses are compromised _____

24. Infection that causes most maxillary sinusitis cases _____

25. Bacteria traveling within the vascular system _____

26. Transport of infected thrombus/embolus into venous sinus _____

True or False

Assign the statement below as either true or false. For deeper understanding, edit the false statements until they are true.

1. Infection is an invasion by and multiplication of pathogens. _____

2. Most of the body's resident microbiota is bacteria. _____

3. The oral cavity resident microbiota is very different from that of the body. _____

4. Oral pathogen infection by more than one species is *polymicrobial*. _____

5. Odontogenic infections can occur with implant placement or graft surgery. _____

6. Majority of intraoral infections are caused by resident *Streptococcus viridians*. _____

7. Most odontogenic infections are not mixed. _____

8. Most odontogenic infections result initially from increased dental biofilm. _____

9. Virulence factors by pathogens can include bacterial toxins. _____

10. The virulence factors help fight colonization of the pathogen. _____

11. The head and neck bacteria can produce beta-lactamases. _____

12. The beta-lactamases are responsible for resistance to pain medications. _____

13. Beta-lactamases are responsible for any initial tissue damage present. _____

14. Careful use of antimicrobials includes using them for every infection. _____

15. Some odontogenic infections can be secondary to tonsillar ones. _____

16. An abscess can feel fluctuant with palpitation. _____

17. An abscess can only be an acute finding. _____

18. Suppuration can be possibly noted on the surface of the fistula's stoma. _____

19. The alveolar process with infection will break down at its thickest part. _____

20. A pustule can only be found extraorally. _____

21. Cellulitis can be noted with firm swelling that feels doughy to indurated. _____

22. Extraoral infections can result in the surface skin having severe scarring. ____

23. Cellulitis is treated by systemic antibiotics and removal of infection cause. _____

24. Osteomyelitis of the jaw is mostly secondary to a periodontal abscess. _____

25. Osteomyelitis of the jaw mainly occurs in the maxillae. _____

26. The sequestrum acts as a reservoir for continuing infection. _____

27. Paresthesia with heaviness may develop with osteomyelitis. _____

28. A perforation may occur in the wall of the sinus with infection. _____

29. Skin over infected sinus will feel cold with palpation. _____

30. Cavernous sinus thrombosis may cause damage to the abducens. _____

Table Completion

Fill in the rest of the table from the indicated textbook table

Table 12.1 Clinical Presentations of Orofacial Abscesses

Clinical Presentation of Lesion	Teeth and Associated Periodontium Region Most Commonly Involved
Maxillary vestibule	
Penetration of nasal floor	
Nasolabial region	
Palate	
Perforation into maxillary sinus	
Buccal mucosal surface	
Mandibular vestibule	
Submental region	
Sublingual region	
Submandibular region	

Table 12.2 Clinical Presentations of Orofacial Cellulitis

Clinical Presentation of Lesion	Space Involved	Teeth and Associated Periodontium Region Most Commonly Involved in Infection
Infraorbital, zygomatic, and buccal regions		
Posterior border of mandible		
Submental region		
Unilateral submandibular region		
Bilateral submandibular region		
Lateral cervical region		

CASE STUDY 1

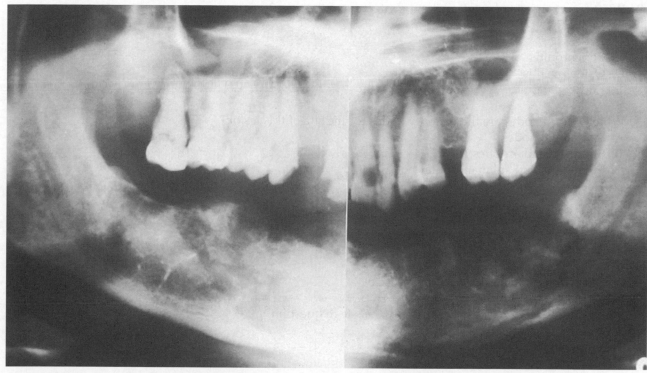

(Courtesy Margaret J. Fehrenbach, RDH, MS.)

Patient	Male, 48 years old
Chief Complaint	*"The bottom of my mouth is bleeding and I have pins-and-needles feeling in my entire lower lip since my surgery."*
Background and/or Patient History	Rock band manager Surgical removal of mandibular dentition for implant preparation Patient has not stopped smoking/chewing tobacco as requested Frequent alcoholic beverages Medications: Narcotic pain medication, Antibiotic, Antiseptic oral rinse
Current Findings	Visiting office of record as follow-up before prosthesis appointments will begin Admits to not performing homecare recommended by local hospital attending oral surgeon Current intraoral examination: bone damage within mandibular alveolar process Current extraoral examination: hemorrhaging with paresthesia of entire lower lip

*Uses Integrated National Board Dental Examination format as determined by the Joint Commission on National Dental Examinations by American Dental Association. Figures courtesy Margaret J. Fehrenbach, RDH, MS.

169

1. Why does bone damage of this kind happen mainly within the mandible?
   A. Thicker cortical plates and increased vascularization
   B. Thinner cortical plates and reduced vascularization
   C. Thicker cortical plates and reduced vascularization
   D. Thinner cortical plates and increased vascularization

2. What term is used to best describe the infection of the bone?
   A. Cellulitis
   B. Abscess
   C. Pericoronitis
   D. Osteomyelitis
   E. Ludwig angina

3. Which lymph nodes are the primary nodes for the site of this lesion?
   A. Submental nodes
   B. Submandibular nodes
   C. Submental and submandibular nodes
   D. Deep cervical nodes

4. Which muscle forms the patient's floor of the mouth?
   A. Zygomaticus major muscle
   B. Mylohyoid muscle
   C. Omohyoid muscle
   D. Superior pharyngeal constrictor muscle

5. Which arteries are most likely to supply the site in question?
   A. Inferior labial artery
   B. Submental artery
   C. Occipital artery
   D. Middle meningeal artery

6. What landmark of the mandible helps the clinician to ascertain information on the patient's paresthesia of the lower lip?
   A. Mandibular foramen
   B. Mental foramen
   C. Internal oblique line
   D. External oblique line

7. What facial landmark separates the lower lip from the chin on the patient?
   A. Nasolabial fold
   B. Glabella
   C. Labiomental groove
   D. Vermilion border

8. Which of the following nerves could also be directly damaged noting the location of the patient's paresthesia?
   A. (Long) buccal nerve
   B. Posterior superior alveolar nerve
   C. Masseter nerve
   D. Mental nerve

9. When the previous dental office anesthetized his mandibular arch before surgery, he felt a kind of "shock," which is commonly due to a(n)
   A. anterior middle superior alveolar local anesthetic block.
   B. Gow-Gates mandibular local anesthetic block.
   C. (long) buccal local anesthetic block.
   D. inferior alveolar local anesthetic block.

10. What bone of the patient articulates with the facial bone involved in the bony damage allowing the patient to open his mouth during the examination?
    A. Sphenoid
    B. Cranial
    C. Facial
    D. Hyoid

CASE STUDY 2

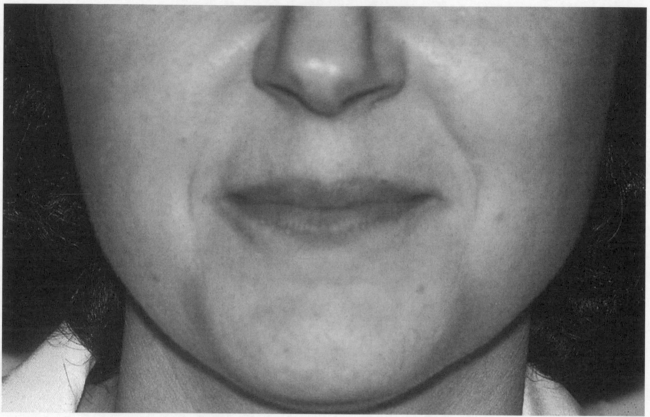

(Courtesy of Margaret J. Fehrenbach, RDH, MS.)

Patient	Female, 59 years old
Chief Complaint	*"My mouth feels like cotton and my jaws are achy. Plus my front tooth has darkened."*
Background and/or Patient History	Retired social worker Osteoarthritis Depression Medications: NSAIDs, Antidepressant
Current Findings	Patient of record is visiting office for a 6-month appointment Past record of hyposalivation with xerostomia due to medication No occlusal evaluation performed due to patient concerns Current extraoral examination: enlarged cheeks with notation of nightly clenching of teeth with morning jaw ache Current intraoral examination: darkened permanent maxillary right central incisor Periodontal examination: slight to moderate mobility of posterior teeth

1. Which areas of the mouth must be palpated to evaluate salivary gland function?
   A. Parotid duct on each buccal mucosa of the cheek
   B. Parotid duct on the buccal mucosa and submandibular duct on the floor of the mouth
   C. Submandibular duct in the mandibular vestibule of the buccal mucosa
   D. Parotid duct on the buccal mucosa as well as submandibular and sublingual ducts on the floor of the mouth

2. Which salivary gland produces the most saliva for this patient?
   A. Parotid gland
   B. Submandibular gland
   C. von Ebner glands
   D. Sublingual gland

3. What is the efferent nerve supply for the submandibular salivary gland?
   A. Glossopharyngeal nerve
   B. Facial nerve
   C. Cervical ganglion
   D. Trigeminal nerve

4. Which of the following bones form a joint that may be affected by the patient's bone disorder?
   A. Parietal and occipital bones
   B. Maxillary and palatine bones
   C. Temporal bone and mandible
   D. Occipital bone and mandible
   E. Maxillary bone and mandible

5. What nerves may be involved in the ache she feels in her jaw?
   A. Chorda tympani
   B. Buccal branch of the facial nerve
   C. Maxillary division of the trigeminal nerve
   D. Mandibular division of the trigeminal nerve

6. What probably has caused the patient's firmly enlarged cheeks?
   A. Overuse of the masseter muscle
   B. Underuse of the temporomandibular ligament
   C. Excess fluid in the synovial cavities
   D. Excess lymph in the disc of the joint

7. Which of the following lymph nodes drain the periodontium associated with the darkened tooth?
   A. Buccal nodes
   B. Submandibular nodes
   C. Submental nodes
   D. Deep parotid nodes

8. Which of the following veins drain the periodontium associated with the darkened tooth?
   A. Superficial temporal vein
   B. Posterior superior alveolar vein
   C. Incisive vein
   D. Mylohyoid vein

9. If there would be further dental treatment on the darkened tooth, which nerve MUST be anesthetized?
   A. Inferior alveolar nerve
   B. Posterior superior alveolar nerve
   C. Mental nerve
   D. Anterior superior alveolar nerve

10. Which local anesthetic blocks could be used to anesthetize the darkened tooth if further dental work were expected?
   A. Posterior superior alveolar block
   B. Middle superior alveolar block
   C. Infraorbital block
   D. Greater palatine block

CASE STUDY 3

Patient	Female, 7 years old
Chief Complaint	*"I burned the top of my mouth—oww—from hot pizza last night!"*
Background and/or Patient History	First grade student Likes using the computer
Current Findings	Patient of record missed the last 6-month appointment due to sore throat Current intraoral examination: enlarged bilateral tonsils near fauces, small superficial ulceration on anterior hard palate, fair homecare level, permanent first molars have enamel sealants

1. Which nerves are involved in the discomfort possibly felt by the patient due to the thermal burn?
   A. Posterior superior alveolar nerve
   B. Lesser palatine nerve
   C. Incisive nerve
   D. Nasopalatine nerves
   E. Anterior superior alveolar nerve

2. Which bone(s) underlie(s) the thermal burn when gently palpated during the intraoral examination?
   A. Palatine bones
   B. Zygomatic bone
   C. Maxillae
   D. Maxillae and palatine bones

3. Which unique intraoral landmark is nearby or within the thermal burn area?
   A. Parotid papilla
   B. Incisive papilla
   C. Retromolar pad
   D. Maxillary tuberosity

4. Which tonsils are involved in the enlargement noted during the examination?
   A. Lingual tonsil
   B. Palatine tonsils
   C. Pharyngeal tonsil
   D. Tubal tonsil

5. Which group of lymph nodes may be palpable during the extraoral examination because the patient has enlarged tonsils?
   A. Superior deep cervical nodes
   B. Submandibular nodes
   C. Submental nodes
   D. Mandibular nodes

6. Which specific lymph nodes may be palpable due to the enlarged tonsils?
   A. Jugulo-omohyoid nodes
   B. Occipital nodes
   C. Jugulodigastric nodes
   D. Auricular nodes

7. When the patient tried to chew the pizza, which muscles were mainly used?
   A. Temporalis muscle
   B. Epicranial muscle
   C. Mentalis muscle
   D. Risorius muscle
   E. Platysma muscle

8. Which muscle helps keep the pizza in the correct position in the mouth during chewing?
   A. Masseter muscle
   B. Buccinator muscle
   C. Risorius muscle
   D. Medial pterygoid muscle

9. Which nerve innervates the muscles that are mainly involved in chewing the pizza?
   A. Facial nerve
   B. Glossopharyngeal nerve
   C. Trigeminal nerve
   D. Abducens nerve

10. Pressure upon examination of the ulcerated area causes the patient to frown, contracting which muscles?
    A. Zygomaticus minor muscle
    B. Corrugator supercilii muscle
    C. Risorius muscle
    D. Zygomaticus major muscle

CASE STUDY 4

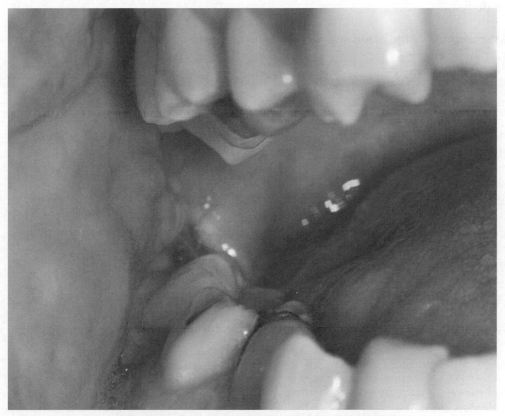

(Courtesy of Margaret J. Fehrenbach, RDH, MS.)

Patient	Male, 32 years old
Chief Complaint	*"My breath feels bad and my lower jaw feels really sore on the left side."*
Background and/or Patient History	Lawyer at downtown firm Height: 5 feet, 9 inches (1.75 metres) Weight: 248 pounds (112.5 kilograms) Blood Pressure: 148/98 High blood pressure diagnosis Medications: Diuretic, Ibuprofen Smokes cigars on weekends No exercise and enjoys fast food
Current Findings	Last appointment 5 years ago before emergency appointment today Current intraoral examination: pericoronal inflammation around partially erupted permanent mandibular left third molar, older amalgam restorations, several broken composite restorations, halitosis with coated tongue Current periodontal examination: severe deposits throughout with moderate levels of gingival bleeding

1. Which lymph nodes listed below drain the site of the oral inflammation?
   A. Submandibular nodes
   B. Mandibular nodes
   C. Buccal nodes
   D. Malar nodes

2. Which arteries provide the blood supply to the site of the oral inflammation?
   A. Inferior labial artery
   B. Inferior alveolar artery
   C. Posterior superior alveolar artery
   D. Retromandibular artery

3. Which nerves could be involved in the discomfort at the site of the oral inflammation?
   A. Mental nerve
   B. (Long) buccal nerve
   C. Incisive nerve
   D. Posterior superior alveolar nerve

4. Which muscle is contracted when the patient sticks out his tongue during the examination?
   A. Pharyngeal constrictor muscles
   B. Hyoglossus muscle
   C. Genioglossus muscle
   D. Styloglossus muscle

5. When the patient brushes his tongue, as directed later during an oral homecare discussion, which nerve feels the sensation?
   A. Posterior superior alveolar nerve
   B. Lingual nerve
   C. Mental nerve
   D. Inferior alveolar nerve

6. Which nerve must be anesthetized to extract the involved tooth, if warranted?
   A. Posterior superior alveolar nerve
   B. Middle superior alveolar nerve
   C. Greater palatine nerve
   D. Inferior alveolar nerve

7. If the involved tooth is extracted, from which bone and its process would the extraction take place?
   A. Maxillary bone and zygomatic process
   B. Mandible and coronoid process
   C. Zygomatic bone and maxillary process
   D. Mandible and alveolar process

8. If the inflammatory process progresses and becomes an infection, which of the following locations of an abscess presentation would be most likely?
   A. Palate
   B. Buccal space
   C. Submental space
   D. Sublingual space
   E. Submandibular space

9. If the spaces associated with the involved tooth were to undergo cellulitis, into which location could the infection travel?
   A. Unilateral zygomatic region
   B. Cavernous sinus
   C. Retropharyngeal space
   D. Maxillary sinus

10. If the patient needs to take pain medication, which muscle will help close off the nasopharynx when he swallows it?
    A. Genioglossus muscle
    B. Inferior pharyngeal constrictor muscle
    C. Hyoglossus muscle
    D. Muscle of the uvula

CASE STUDY 5

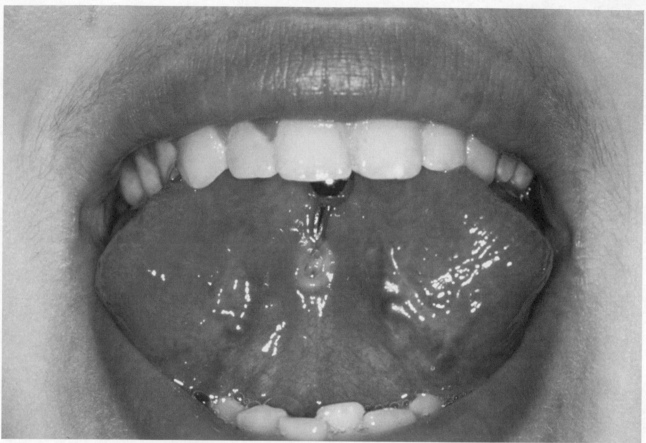

(Courtesy of Margaret J. Fehrenbach, RDH, MS.)

Patient	Male, 27 years old
Chief Complaint	*"My tongue is sore around the stud and there is a bad taste in my mouth..."*
Background and/or Patient History	Microbrewer Medications: Aspirin, Alcohol mouthwash
Current Findings	New patient emergency appointment Regular care until recently moved from childhood home No restorations or caries present Past history orthodontic therapy but never wore recommended retainer Temperature: 98.6 F Current extraoral examination: Adjoining region slight lymphadenopathy Current intraoral examination: suppuration around tongue-piercing jewelry from localized infection Current periodontal examination: moderate deposits with slight to moderate gingival bleeding

1. In what part of the tongue is the localized lesion located?
   A. Base
   B. Body
   C. Lateral
   D. Apex

2. Which of the following infections could occur secondarily in this patient due to the present situation with his tongue?
   A. Gingival abscess
   B. Ludwig angina
   C. Maxillary sinus infection
   D. Pericoronitis

3. If severe bleeding occurred when the patient had his tongue pierced, which of the following structures were possibly involved?
   A. Carotid arteries and veins
   B. Lingual frenum
   C. Lingual arteries and veins
   D. Carotid arteries and veins and lingual frenum

4. Which of the following spaces can be initially involved in the localized tongue infection if it progresses?
   A. Buccal space
   B. Canine space
   C. Submandibular space
   D. Submasseteric space

5. Which lymph nodes would be initially involved due to this localized tongue infection?
   A. Submandibular nodes
   B. Retroauricular nodes
   C. Mandibular nodes
   D. Retropharyngeal nodes

6. If the patient has a serious secondary infection occur later, what symptoms would be present that would be of diagnostic level?
   A. Nasal drainage
   B. Hoarseness
   C. Bleeding at the site
   D. Difficulty swallowing

7. What muscles mainly allow him to flatten his tongue to show off his tongue piercing?
   A. Transverse and vertical muscles
   B. Omohyoid muscle
   C. Genioglossus muscle
   D. Hyoglossus muscle

8. Which lymph nodes would be secondary nodes for the localized tongue infection if it progressed?
   A. Submandibular nodes
   B. Submental nodes
   C. Superior deep cervical nodes
   D. Retropharyngeal nodes

9. If he accidentally swallowed the tongue jewelry when it was being placed, what pharyngeal muscle(s) would help him move it toward the esophagus?
   A. Genioglossus muscle
   B. Infrahyoid muscles
   C. Digastric muscle
   D. Pharyngeal constrictor muscles

10. What is the sensory innervation for the part of the tongue involved in soreness?
   A. Abducent nerve
   B. Facial nerve
   C. Glossopharyngeal nerve
   D. Lingual nerve

CASE STUDY 6

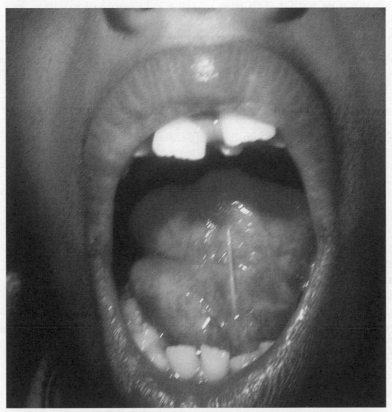

(Courtesy of Margaret J. Fehrenbach, RDH, MS.)

Patient	Female, 35 years old
Chief Complaint	*"Right before I eat, the bottom of my mouth seems to grow larger!"*
Background and/or Patient History	Registered nurse Height: 5 feet, 10 inches (1.78 metres) Weight: 125 pounds (56.7 kilograms) Blood Pressure: 95/75 Marathon runner Allergy to pollen Medications: Allergy medications, Alcohol mouthwash
Current Findings	Referred by local clinic for initial appointment Current intraoral and extraoral examinations: unilateral salivary gland enlargement with palpable stone Current periodontal examination: excellent dental health with crowded dentition Low caries risk

1. Which of the following statements concerning salivary glands is correct?
   A. Salivary glands are endocrine glands.
   B. Salivary glands are controlled by the somatic nervous system.
   C. Salivary glands have both minor and minor glands.
   D. Salivary glands cannot be palpated during an extraoral examination.

2. Which of the following salivary glands is most commonly involved in salivary stone formation?
   A. Parotid gland
   B. Submandibular gland
   C. Sublingual gland
   D. Minor glands

3. If the stone were removed during surgery, which nerve may be injured?
   A. Inferior alveolar nerve
   B. Lingual nerve
   C. Auriculotemporal nerve
   D. Facial nerve

4. Which of the following glands is located posterior to the gland involved in this lesion?
   A. Parotid gland
   B. Lacrimal gland
   C. Sublingual gland
   D. Thyroid gland

5. What muscle listed below does both the smaller and deeper lobe of the involved gland wrap around?
   A. Genioglossus muscle
   B. Omohyoid muscle
   C. Digastric muscle
   D. Mylohyoid muscle

6. What nerve and its efferent (parasympathetic) fibers innervate the involved gland?
   A. Chorda tympani
   B. Inferior alveolar
   C. Lingual
   D. Mental

7. Into which lymph nodes does the involved gland directly drain?
   A. Submental nodes
   B. Submandibular nodes
   C. Deep parotid nodes
   D. Superficial parotid nodes

8. What type of secretions does the involved gland produce?
   A. Mixed product
   B. Only serous product
   C. Only mucous product
   D. Mainly mucous product

9. What is the intraoral lesion presented by the involved gland?
   A. Mucocele
   B. Pustule
   C. Abscess
   D. Ranula

10. Where does the duct of the involved gland open up within the oral cavity?
    A. Lower lip
    B. Sublingual caruncle
    C. Inner surface of the cheek
    D. Lateral border of tongue

CASE STUDY 7

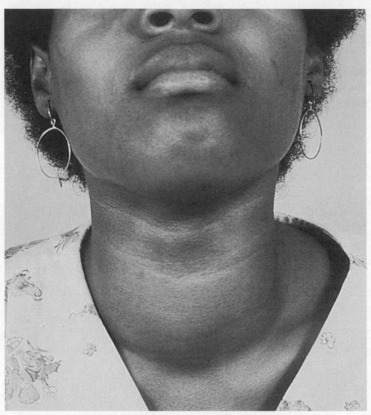

(Courtesy of Margaret J. Fehrenbach, RDH, MS.)

Patient	Female, 45 years old
Chief Complaint	*"My neck seems to be getting larger and lumpy in the front."*
Background and/or Patient History	Unemployed office administrator Height: 5 feet, 4 inches (1.63 metres) Weight: 226 pounds (102.5 kilograms) Hypothyroidism Major recent weight gain Medications: Used to take thyroid medication but lost drug coverage
Current Findings	Uncomfortable talking about lack of care since last appointment over 5 years Current extraoral examination: bilateral enlargement of thyroid gland inferior and posterior to body of mandible Current intraoral examination: oral health is compromised with mucosal ulcerations but only light deposits High caries risk due to enamel erosion from constant diet soda intake

1. The enlargement of the involved gland is considered a
   A. ranula.
   B. mucocele.
   C. goiter.
   D. stone.

2. Into which lymph nodes does the involved gland directly drains
   A. Submental nodes
   B. Submandibular nodes
   C. Superior deep cervical nodes
   D. Inferior deep cervical nodes

3. Which of the following vessels supplies most of the vascularity to the involved gland?
   A. Sublingual arteries
   B. Submental arteries
   C. Facial and lingual arteries
   D. Superior and inferior thyroid arteries

4. Which of the following supplies most of the innervation to the involved gland?
   A. Cervical ganglia
   B. Seventh cranial nerve
   C. Chorda tympani nerve
   D. Ninth cranial nerve

5. Into which fascia or fascial space is the involved gland mainly encased?
   A. Visceral fascia
   B. Submandibular space
   C. Retropharyngeal space
   D. Carotid sheath

6. In which cervical compartment is the involved gland located?
   A. Vertebral compartment
   B. Visceral compartment
   C. Vascular compartments
   D. Vertebral and visceral compartments

7. Which type of fasciae encases the involved gland of the patient?
   A. Visceral fascia
   B. Vertebral fascia
   C. Investing fascia
   D. Pterygoid fascia

8. Which of the following is also in the same cervical compartment as the involved gland?
   A. Spinal cord
   B. Carotid sheath
   C. Parotid salivary gland
   D. Hyoid bone

9. Which of the following is known to be part of the body of the mandible?
   A. Alveolar process of the mandible
   B. Alveoli for the mandibular teeth
   C. Facial and lingual cortical plates
   D. Angle of the mandible

10. Which of the following is the most superior to the involved gland?
    A. Hyoid bone
    B. Thyroid cartilage
    C. Superior thyroid notch
    D. Larynx

CASE STUDY 8

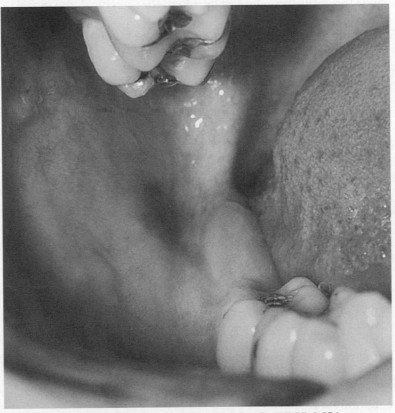

(Courtesy of Margaret J. Fehrenbach, RDH, MS.)

Patient	Male, 22 years old
Chief Complaint	*"There is a large dark bump in my mouth where they did some dental work!"*
Background and/or Patient History	College student in art studies
Current Findings	Referred from downtown emergency clinic after recent restorative to permanent mandibular second molar and extraoral examination sinuses superior to posterior part of upper jaw to check on pressure from slight common cold Current intraoral examination: flat bluish lesion on medial surface of mandibular ramus with short duration with slight discomfort, slight caries risk States homecare has improved since last appointment Slight caries risk

1. Which of the following is considered a definition of the patient's lesion?
   A. Small amount of blood escapes into the surrounding tissue and clots.
   B. Narrowing and blockage of the arteries by a buildup of plaque.
   C. Large amounts of blood that escape into the surrounding tissue without clotting
   D. Foreign material or thrombus traveling in the blood that can block the vessel.

2. Which of the following blood vessels or its branches may be involved in this lesion?
   A. Facial artery
   B. Inferior alveolar artery
   C. Posterior superior alveolar artery
   D. Mental artery

3. When incorrectly giving the local anesthetic block associated with this lesion, what other lesion can occur that mainly involves the seventh cranial nerve?
   A. Transient facial paralysis
   B. Extraoral hematoma
   C. Paresthesia
   D. Lingual shock

4. If the local anesthetic block associated with this lesion is given correctly, which of the following is considered the most reliable indicator of success?
   A. Numbness of the tongue
   B. No discomfort during procedures
   C. Tingling of the floor of the mouth
   D. Numbness of lower lip

5. Which of the following was the recommended target site for the local anesthetic block associated with this lesion?
   A. Anterior border of the ramus
   B. Anterior to the mental foramen
   C. Pterygomandibular space
   D. Anteromedial border of the condylar neck

6. Which of the following is included in a description of the mandibular ramus?
   A. Stout flat plate that rises up from the angle
   B. Posterior border terminates in the coronoid process
   C. Anterior border forms a convex posterior curve of the coronoid notch
   D. Posterior border becomes the external oblique line

7. Which of the following is included in a correct definition of medial?
   A. Part that is directed toward the posterior
   B. Front of an area but not back of an area
   C. Area closer to the midsagittal plane
   D. Area farther way from the midsagittal plane

8. If the floor of the examined sinuses is the alveolar process, what is the roof?
   A. Maxillary tuberosity
   B. Lateral wall of nasal cavity
   C. Maxillary premolars and molars
   D. Orbital floor

9. Into which of the following drain the examined sinuses?
   A. Superior nasal meatus
   B. External acoustic meatus
   C. Middle nasal meatus
   D. Inferior nasal meatus

10. If the patient would have had an infection in the sinuses at the last appointment, which of the following could have been directly involved?
    A. Foul discharge from internal acoustic meatus
    B. Perforation possibly spreading infection
    C. Tender and cool skin over sinuses
    D. Thinning of sinus walls on radiographs

NOTES

NOTES

Head Regions

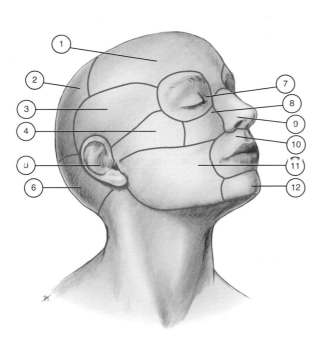

1
2
3
4
5
6
7
8
9
10
11
12

Neck Regions and Cervical Muscles

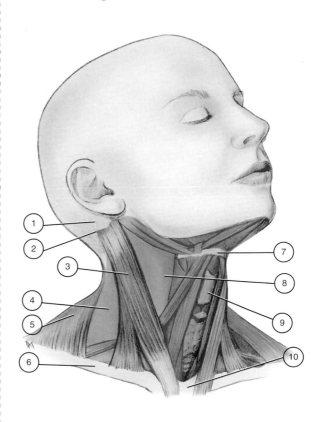

1
2
3
4
5
6
7
8
9
10

Cranial Bones—Lateral View

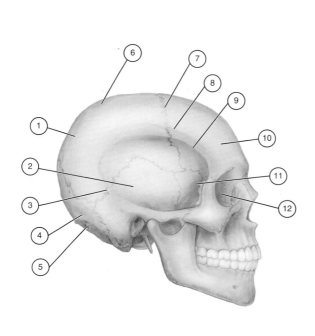

1
2
3
4
5
6
7
8
9
10
11
12

Facial Bones—Anterior View

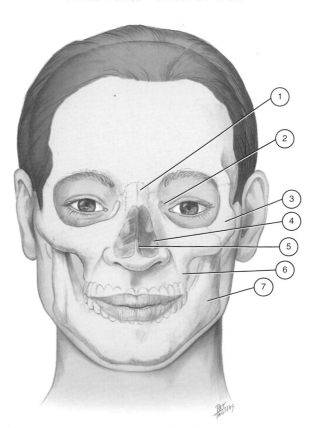

1
2
3
4
5
6
7

Neck Regions and Cervical Muscles

1. Mastoid process of the temporal bone

2. Superior nuchal line of the occipital bone

3. Sternocleidomastoid muscle

4. Posterior cervical triangle

5. Trapezius muscle

6. Clavicle

7. Hyoid bone

8. Anterior cervical triangle

9. Thyroid cartilage

10. Sternum

Head Regions

1. Frontal region

2. Parietal region

3. Temporal region

4. Zygomatic region

5. Auricular region

6. Occipital region

7. Orbital region

8. Infraorbital region

9. Nasal region

10. Oral region

11. Buccal region

12. Mental region

Facial Bones—Anterior View

1. Nasal bone

2. Lacrimal bone

3. Zygomatic bone

4. Inferior nasal concha

5. Vomer

6. Maxilla

7. Mandible

Cranial Bones—Lateral View

1. Parietal bone

2. Temporal bone

3. Squamosal suture

4. Occipital bone

5. Lambdoidal suture

6. Sagittal suture

7. Coronal suture

8. Superior temporal line

9. Inferior temporal line

10. Frontal bone

11. Sphenoid bone

12. Ethmoid bone

External Skull—Inferior View-A

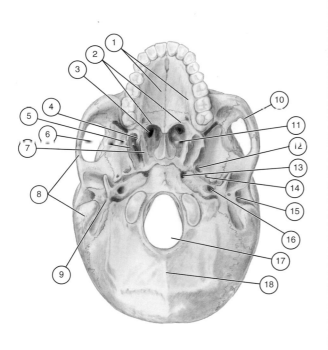

External Skull—Inferior View-B

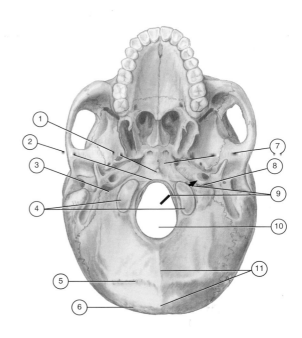

External Skull—Inferior View-C

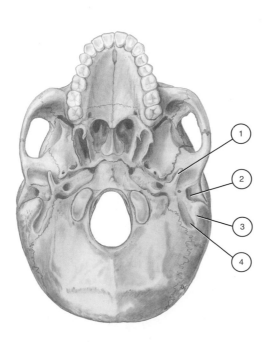

External Skull—Posteror View

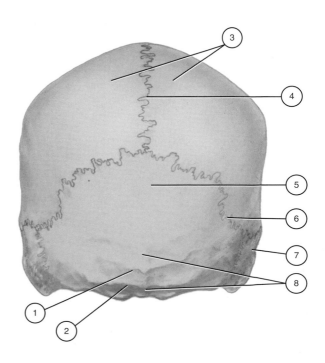

External Skull—Inferior View-B

1. Pharyngeal tubercle

2. Basion

3. Jugular notch of the occipital bone

4. Occipital condyles

5. Inferior nuchal line

6. Superior nuchal line

7. Basilar part of the occipital bone

8. Jugular foramen

9. Hypoglossal canal

10. Foramen magnum

11. External occipital protuberance

External Skull—Inferior View-A

1. Maxillae
2. Palatine bones
3. Posterior nasal aperture
4. Hamulus of the medial plate
5. Pterygoid fossa
6. Lateral pterygoid plate of the sphenoid bone
7. Medial pterygoid plate of the sphenoid bone
8. Temporal bone
9. Stylomastoid foramen
10. Zygomatic bone
11. Vomer
12. Foramen ovale
13. Foramen lacerum
14. Foramen spinosum
15. External acoustic meatus
16. Carotid canal
17. Foramen magnum
18. Occipital bone

External Skull—Posteror View

1. Superior nuchal line

2. Occipital condyles

3. Parietal bones

4. Sagittal suture

5. Occipital bone

6. Lambdoidal suture

7. Temporal bone

8. External occipital protuberance

External Skull—Inferior View-C

1. Styloid process

2. External acoustic meatus

3. Mastoid process

4. Mastoid notch

Internal Skull—Superior View

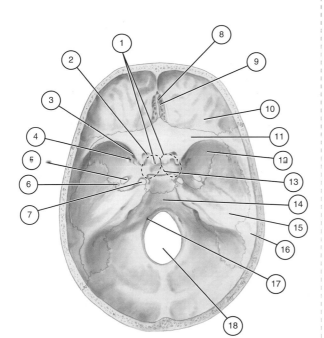

1
2
3
4
5
6
7
8
9
10
11
12
13
14
15
16
17
18

Orbit—Anterior View

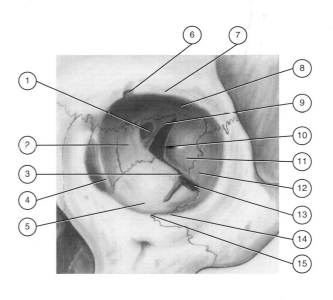

1
?
3
4
5
6
7
8
9
10
11
12
13
14
15

Nasal Cavity—Lateral Wall

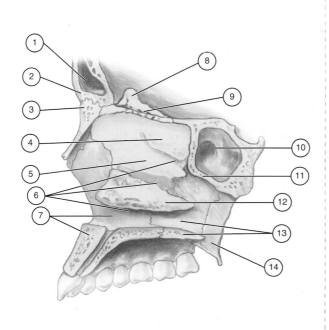

1
2
3
4
5
6
7
8
9
10
11
12
13
14

Maxillae—Anterior View

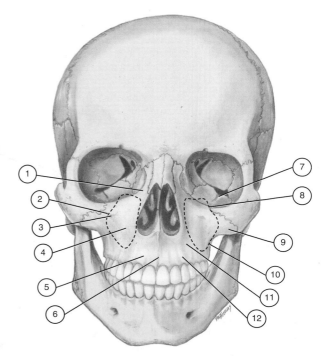

1
2
3
4
5
6
7
8
9
10
11
12

Orbit—Anterior View

1. Optic canal
2. Ethmoid bone
3. Palatine bone
4. Lacrimal bone
5. Maxilla
6. Supraorbital notch
7. Supraorbital rim
8. Frontal bone
9. Lesser wing of the sphenoid bone
10. Superior orbital fissure
11. Greater wing of the sphenoid bone
12. Zygomatic bone
13. Inferior orbital fissure
14. Infraorbital rim
15. Zygomaticomaxillary suture

Internal Skull—Superior View

1. Sphenoidal sinuses of the sphenoid bone location
2. Optical canal
3. Superior orbital fissure
4. Foramen rotundum
5. Foramen ovale
6. Foramen spinosum
7. Carotid canal
8. Crista galli of the ethmoid bone
9. Cribriform plate of the ethmoid bone
10. Frontal bone
11. Lesser wing of the sphenoid bone
12. Greater wing of the sphenoid bone
13. Body of the sphenoid bone
14. Occipital bone
15. Temporal bone
16. Parietal bone
17. Hypoglossal canal
18. Foramen magnum

Maxillae—Anterior View

1. Frontal process of the maxilla
2. Location of the maxillary sinus
3. Infraorbital foramen
4. Body of the maxilla
5. Alveolar process of the maxilla
6. Intermaxillary suture
7. Infraorbital sulcus
8. Infraorbital rim
9. Zygomatic process of the maxilla
10. Location of maxillary sinus
11. Canine fossa
12. Canine eminence

Nasal Cavity—Lateral Wall

1. Frontal sinus
2. Frontal bone
3. Nasal bone
4. Superior nasal concha of the ethmoid bone
5. Middle nasal conchae of the ethmoid bone
6. Nasal meatuses: superior, middle, inferior
7. Maxilla
8. Crista galli of the ethmoid bone
9. Cribriform plate of the ethmoid bone
10. Sphenoidal sinus of the sphenoid bone
11. Sphenoid bone
12. Inferior nasal concha
13. Palatine bone
14. Medial pterygoid plate of the sphenoid bone

Maxilla—Lateral View

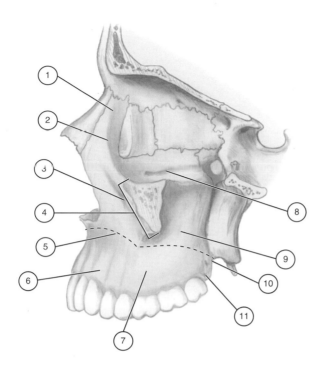

Mandible—Lateral View

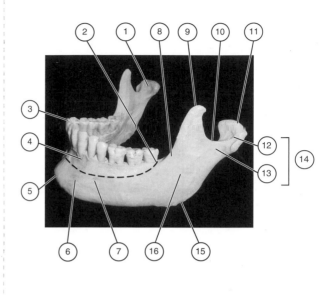

(Courtesy Margaret J. Fehrenbach, RDH, MS)

Mandible—Medial View

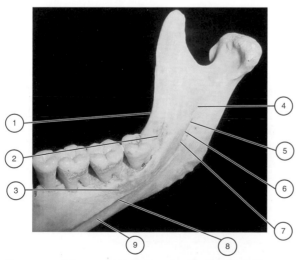

Courtesy Margaret J. Fehrenbach, RDH, MS

Hard Palate—Inferior View

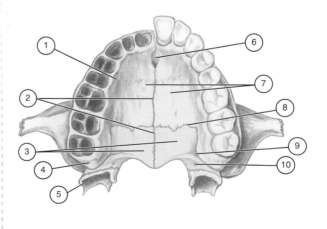

Mandible—Lateral View

1. Pterygoid fovea
2. External oblique line
3. Mandibular teeth
4. Alveolar process of the mandible
5. Mental protuberance
6. Body of the mandible
7. Mental foramen
8. Coronoid notch
9. Coronoid process
10. Mandibular notch
11. Articulating surface of the mandibular condyle
12. Neck of the mandibular condyle
13. Mandibular condyle
14. Condyloid process
15. Angle of the mandible
16. Mandibular ramus

Maxilla—Lateral View

1. Frontal process of the maxilla
2. Infraorbital rim
3. Infraorbital foramen
4. Zygomatic process of the maxilla
5. Canine fossa
6. Canine eminence
7. Alveolar process of the maxilla
8. Infraorbital sulcus
9. Body of the maxilla
10. Posterior superior alveolar foramina
11. Maxillary tuberosity

Hard Palate—Inferior View

1. Alveolar process of the maxilla
2. Median palatine suture
3. Horizontal plates of the palatine bones
4. Maxillary tuberosity
5. Sphenoid bone
6. Incisive foramen
7. Palatine processes of the maxillae
8. Transverse palatine suture
9. Greater palatine foramen
10. Lesser palatine foramen

Mandible—Medial View

1. Coronoid notch
2. Retromolar triangle
3. Sublingual fossa
4. Mandibular ramus
5. Mandibular foramen
6. Lingula
7. Mylohyoid groove
8. Mylohyoid line
9. Submandibular fossa

Temporomandibular Joint—Sagittal Section

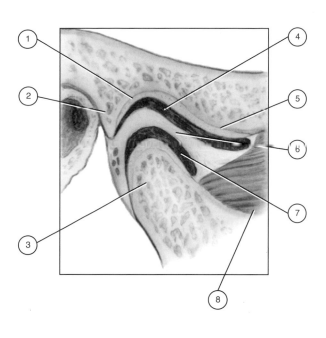

Paranasal Sinuses

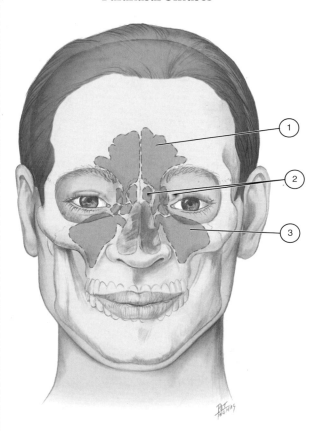

Skull Fossae and Borders—Oblique Lateral View

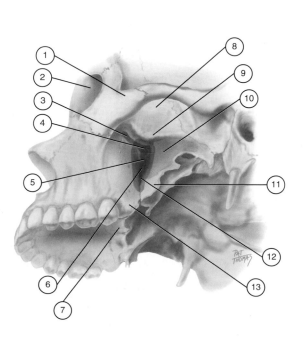

Muscles of Facial Expression—Frontal View

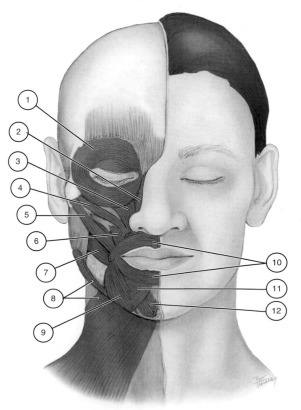

Paranasal Sinuses

1. Frontal sinus of the frontal bone

2. Ethmoidal sinuses of the ethmoid bone

3. Maxillary sinus of the maxilla

Temporomandibular Joint—Sagittal Section

1. Articular fossa

2. Postglenoid process

3. Mandibular condyle

4. Upper synovial cavity

5. Articular eminence

6. Joint disc of the temporomandibular joint

7. Lower synovial cavity

8. Lateral pterygoid muscle

Muscles of Facial Expression—Frontal View

1. Orbicularis oculi muscle

2. Levator labii superioris alaeque nasi muscle

3. Levator labii superioris muscle

4. Zygomaticus minor muscle

5. Zygomaticus major muscle

6. Levator anguli oris muscle

7. Buccinator muscle

8. Platysma muscle

9. Depressor anguli oris muscle

10. Orbicularis oris muscle

11. Depressor labii inferioris muscle

12. Mentalis muscle

Skull Fossae and Borders—Oblique Lateral View

1. Zygomatic arch
2. Orbit
3. Inferior orbital fissure
4. Sphenopalatine foramen
5. Pterygopalatine fossa
6. Pterygomaxillary fissure
7. Palatine bone
8. Temporal fossa
9. Infratemporal crest of greater wing of sphenoid bone
10. Infratemporal fossa
11. Lateral pterygoid plate of the sphenoid bone
12. Pterygopalatine canal
13. Maxillary tuberosity

Muscles of Facial Expression—Lateral View

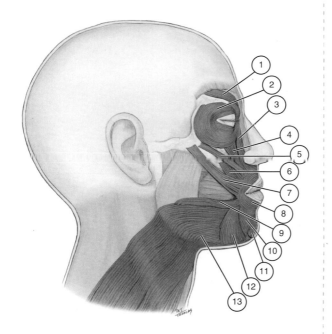

Muscles of Mastication—Lateral View

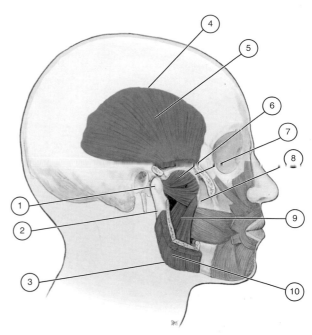

Hyoid Muscles—Anterior View

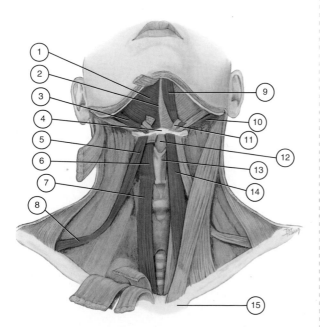

Floor of Oral Cavity with Muscles, Mandible, and Hyoid Bone

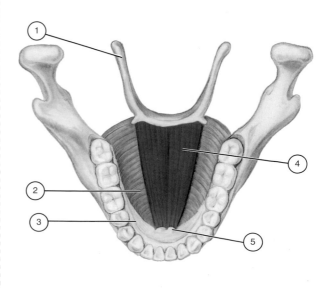

Muscles of Mastication—Lateral View

1. Mandibular condyle
2. Mandibular ramus
3. Angle of the mandible
4. Inferior temporal line
5. Temporalis muscle
6. Lateral pterygoid muscle
7. Sphenoid bone
8. Maxilla
9. Medial pterygoid muscle
10. Masseter muscle

Muscles of Facial Expression—Lateral View

1. Corrugator supercilii muscle
2. Orbicularis oculi muscle
3. Levator labii superioris alaeque nasi muscle
4. Levator labii superioris muscle
5. Zygomaticus minor muscle
6. Levator anguli oris muscle
7. Zygomaticus major muscle
8. Orbicularis oris muscle
9. Risorius muscle
10. Depressor labii inferioris muscle
11. Mentalis muscle
12. Depressor anguli oris muscle
13. Platysma muscle

Floor of Oral Cavity with Muscles, Mandible, and Hyoid Bone

1. Hyoid bone
2. Mylohyoid muscle
3. Medial surface of mandible
4. Geniohyoid muscle
5. Genial tubercles

Hyoid Muscles—Anterior View

1. Mylohyoid muscle
2. Mylohyoid raphe
3. Stylohyoid muscle
4. Hyoid bone
5. Superior belly of the omohyoid muscle
6. Thyrohyoid muscle
7. Sternothyroid muscle
8. Inferior belly of the omohyoid muscle
9. Anterior belly of the digastric muscle
10. Posterior belly of the digastric muscle
11. Intermediate tendon of the digastric muscle
12. Thyrohyoid membrane
13. Thyroid cartilage
14. Sternohyoid muscle
15. Sternum

Tongue With Intrinsic and Extrinsic Muscles—Parasagittal Section—A

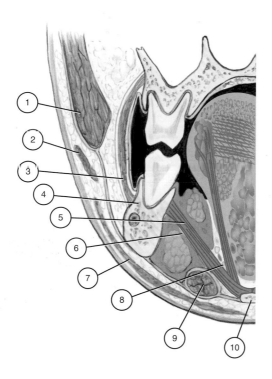

Tongue With Intrinsic and Extrinsic Muscles—Parasagittal Section—B

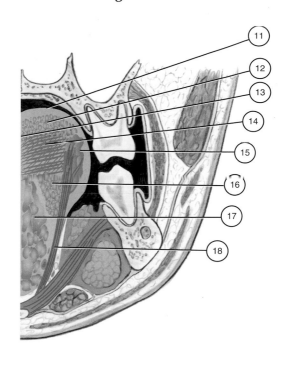

Major Blood Vessels of Head and Neck—Anterior View

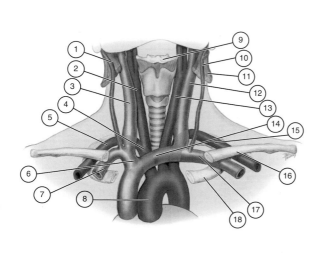

External Carotid Artery—Lateral View

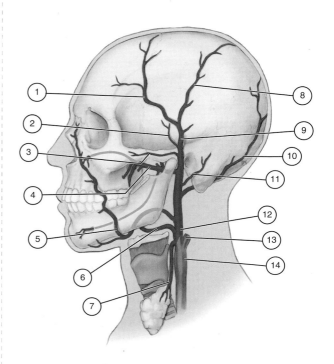

Tongue With Intrinsic and Extrinsic Muscles—
Parasagittal Section—B

11. Tongue epithelium with lingual papillae

12. Superior longitudinal muscle

13. Median septum

14. Styloglossus muscle

15. Inferior longitudinal muscle

16. Genioglossus muscle

17. Hyoglossus muscle

Tongue With Intrinsic and Extrinsic Muscles—
Parasagittal Section—A

1. Masseter muscle

2. Muscles of facial expression

3. Buccinator muscle

4. Mandible

5. Mylohyoid muscle

6. Mylohyoid nerve

7. Platysma muscle

8. Hypoglossal muscle (XIII)

9. Digastric muscle

10. Hyoid bone

External Carotid Artery—Lateral View

1. Frontal branch of superficial temporal artery
2. Middle temporal artery
3. Transverse facial artery
4. Maxillary artery
5. Facial artery
6. Lingual artery
7. Superior thyroid artery
8. Parietal branch of superficial temporal artery
9. Superficial temporal artery
10. Occipital artery
11. Posterior auricular artery
12. External carotid artery
13. Internal carotid artery
14. Common carotid artery

Major Blood Vessels of Head and Neck—
Anterior View

1. Right external jugular vein
2. Right common carotid artery
3. Right internal jugular vein
4. Brachiocephalic artery
5. Right subclavian artery
6. Right brachiocephalic vein
7. Right subclavian vein
8. Aorta
9. Hyoid bone
10. Left external jugular vein
11. Sternocleidomastoid muscle
12. Left internal jugular vein
13. Left common carotid artery
14. Left brachiocephalic vein
15. Left subclavian artery
16. Clavicle
17. Left subclavian vein
18. First rib

Maxillary Artery—Lateral View

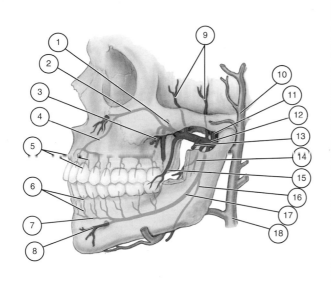

Veins of the Head—Lateral View

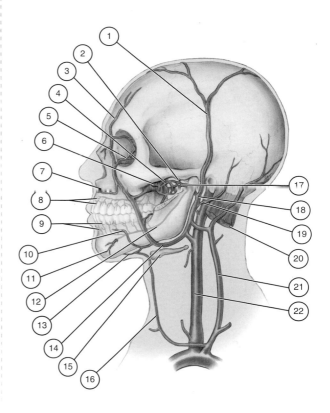

Salivary Glands

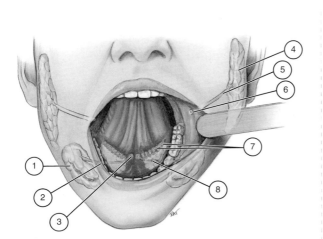

Brain—Sagittal Section

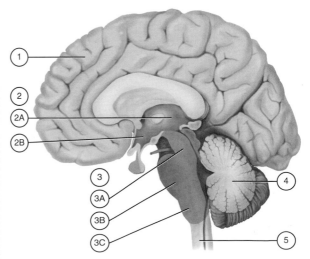

Veins of the Head—Lateral View

1. Superficial temporal vein
2. Middle meningeal vein
3. Supraorbital vein
4. Pterygoid plexus of veins
5. Ophthalmic vein
6. Posterior superior alveolar veins
7. Superior labial vein
8. Alveolar and dental branches of posterior superior alveolar vein
9. Alveolar and dental branches of inferior alveolar vein
10. Inferior labial vein
11. Mental branch of inferior alveolar vein
12. Inferior alveolar vein
13. Submental vein
14. Facial vein
15. Hyoid bone
16. Anterior jugular vein
17. Maxillary vein
18. Retromandibular vein
19. Posterior auricular vein
20. Sternocleidomastoid muscle
21. External jugular vein
22. Internal jugular vein

Maxillary Artery—Lateral View

1. Sphenopalatine artery
2. Infraorbital artery
3. Posterior superior alveolar artery
4. Anterior superior alveolar artery
5. Dental and alveolar branches of superior alveolar artery
6. Dental and alveolar branches of incisive artery
7. Incisive artery
8. Mental artery
9. Deep temporal arteries
10. Superficial temporal artery
11. Middle meningeal artery
12. Maxillary artery
13. Masseteric artery
14. Pterygoid arteries
15. Buccal artery
16. Mylohyoid artery
17. Inferior alveolar artery
18. Left external carotid artery

Brain—Sagittal Section

1. Cerebral hemisphere

2. Diencephalon
   2A. Thalamus
   2B. Hypothalamus

3. Brainstem
   3A. Midbrain
   3B. Pons
   3C. Medulla

4. Cerebellum

5. Spinal cord

Salivary Glands

1. Submandibular salivary gland

2. Submandibular duct

3. Sublingual caruncle

4. Parotid salivary gland

5. Parotid duct

6. Parotid papilla

7. Sublingual ducts

8. Sublingual salivary gland

Cranial Nerves and Internal Skull—Superior View

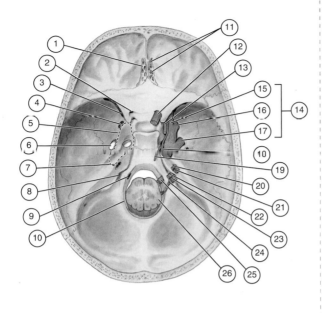

Trigeminal Nerve—Lateral View

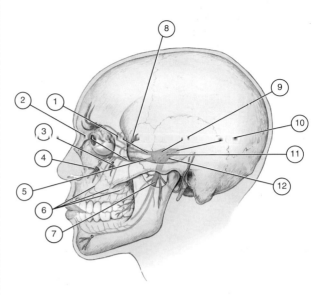

Maxillary Nerve—Lateral View

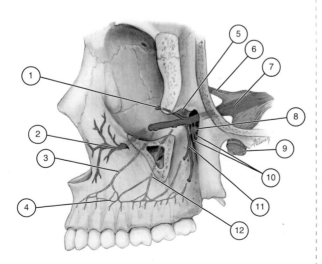

Mandibular Nerve—Lateral View

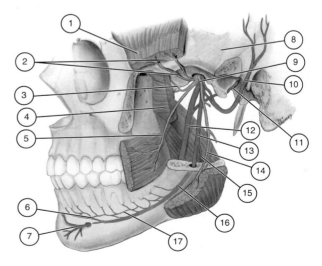

Trigeminal Nerve—Lateral View

1. Ophthalmic division (V_1)
2. Zygomatic nerve
3. Zygomaticofacial nerve
4. Infraorbital nerve
5. Maxillary division (V_2)
6. Superior alveolar nerves
7. Mandibular division (V_3)
8. Zygomaticotemporal nerve
9. Trigeminal ganglion
10. Trigeminal nerve (V)
11. Motor root
12. Sensory root

Cranial Nerves and Internal Skull—Superior View

1. Cribriform plate of the ethmoid bone
2. Optic canal
3. Superior orbital fissure
4. Foramen rotundum
5. Location of cavernous sinus
6. Foramen ovale
7. Internal acoustic meatus
8. Jugular foramen
9. Hypoglossal canal
10. Foramen magnum
11. Olfactory nerve (I) fibers
12. Optic nerve (II)
13. Oculomotor nerve (III)
14. Trigeminal nerve (V)
15. Ophthalmic nerve (V_1)
16. Maxillary nerve (V_2)
17. Mandibular nerve (V_3)
18. Trochlear nerve (IV)
19. Abducens nerve (VI)
20. Facial nerve (VII)
21. Vestibulocochlear nerve (VIII)
22. Glossopharyngeal nerve (IX)
23. Vagus nerve (X)
24. Accessory nerve (XI)
25. Hypoglossal nerve (XII)
26. Spinal cord

Mandibular Nerve—Lateral View

1. Temporalis muscle
2. Anterior and posterior deep temporal nerves
3. Lateral pterygoid nerve
4. Lateral pterygoid muscle
5. Buccal nerve
6. Incisive nerve
7. Mental nerve
8. Location of trigeminal ganglion
9. Mandibular nerve
10. Auriculotemporal nerve
11. Chorda tympani nerve in petrotympanic fissure
12. Lingual nerve
13. Inferior alveolar nerve
14. Masseteric nerve
15. Mylohyoid nerve
16. Inferior alveolar nerve
17. Inferior dental plexus

Maxillary Nerve—Lateral View

1. Zygomatic nerve
2. Infraorbital nerve
3. Anterior superior alveolar nerve
4. Superior dental plexus
5. Inferior orbital fissure
6. Ophthalmic nerve
7. Maxillary nerve
8. Pterygopalatine ganglion
9. Mandibular nerve
10. Greater and lesser palatine nerves
11. Posterior superior alveolar nerve
12. Middle superior alveolar nerve

Lymphatic System

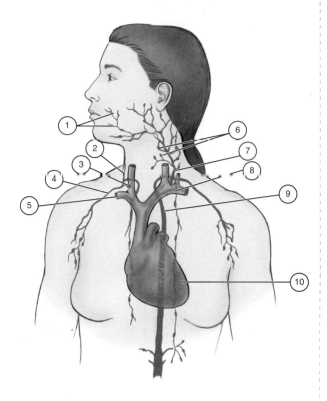

Superficial Lymph Nodes of the Head

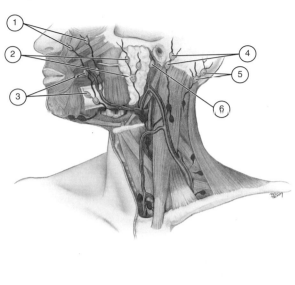

Superficial Cervical Lymph Nodes

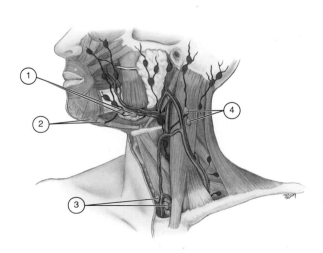

Deep Cervical Lymph Nodes

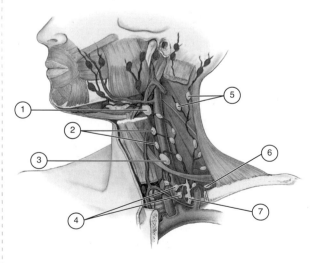

Superficial Lymph Nodes of the Head

1. Facial lymph nodes

2. Superficial parotid lymph nodes

3. Facial lymph nodes

4. Posterior auricular lymph nodes

5. Occipital lymph nodes

6. Anterior auricular lymph nodes

Lymphatic System

1. Facial lymph nodes

2. Right jugular trunk

3. Right lymphatic duct

4. Right subclavian trunk

5. Right subclavian vein

6. Cervical lymph nodes

7. Left jugular trunk

8. Left subclavian trunk

9. Thoracic duct

10. Heart

Deep Cervical Lymph Nodes

1. Jugulodigastric lymph node

2. Superior deep cervical lymph nodes

3. Jugulo-omohyoid lymph node

4. Inferior deep cervical lymph nodes

5. Accessory lymph nodes

6. Supraclavicular lymph node

7. Thoracic duct

Superficial Cervical Lymph Nodes

1. Submandibular lymph nodes

2. Submental lymph nodes

3. Anterior jugular lymph nodes

4. External jugular lymph nodes

Pterygomandibular Space—Transverse Head and Neck Section

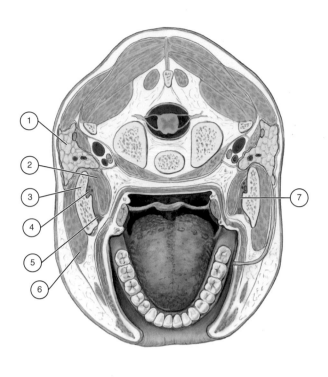

Submandibular and Sublingual Spaces—Frontal Head and Neck Section

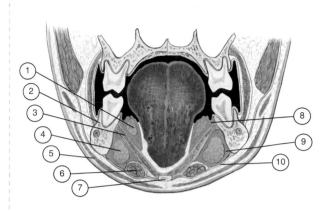

Previsceral and Retropharyngeal Space—Transverse Neck Section

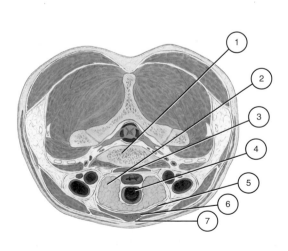

Parapharyngeal and Retropharyngeal Space—Transverse Oral Cavity and Neck Section

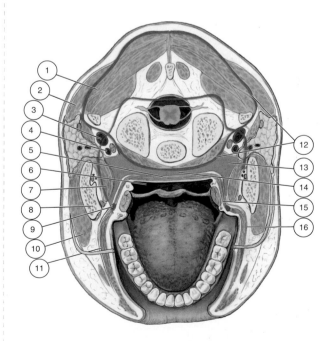

Submandibular and Sublingual Spaces— Frontal Head and Neck Section

1. Sublingual salivary gland

2. Mandible

3. Mylohyoid muscle

4. Submandibular salivary gland

5. Platysma muscle

6. Digastric muscle

7. Hyoid bone

8. Sublingual space

9. Submandibular space

10. Investing fascia

Pterygomandibular Space—Transverse Head and Neck Section

1. Parotid salivary gland

2. Medial pterygoid muscle

3. Mandible

4. Inferior alveolar nerve

5. Lingual nerve

6. Masseter muscle

7. Pterygomandibular space

Parapharyngeal and Retropharyngeal Space— Transverse Oral Cavity and Neck Section

1. Vertebral muscles
2. Sternocleidomastoid muscle
3. Internal jugular vein
4. Internal carotid artery
5. Superior pharyngeal constrictor muscle
6. Pharynx
7. Medial pterygoid muscle
8. Mandible
9. Pterygomandibular raphe
10. Masseter muscle
11. Buccinator muscle
12. Vertebral fascia
13. Parapharyngeal space
14. Retropharyngeal space
15. Buccopharyngeal fascia
16. Buccal space

Previsceral and Retropharyngeal Space— Transverse Neck Section

1. Cervical vertebra with perivertebral space

2. Thyroid gland

3. Retropharyngeal space

4. Trachea

5. Visceral fascia

6. Previsceral space

7. Investing fascia